VOLKER LANGE ■ **Medicynical**
Cartoons from the Daily Routine in Medicine

**VOLKER LANGE**

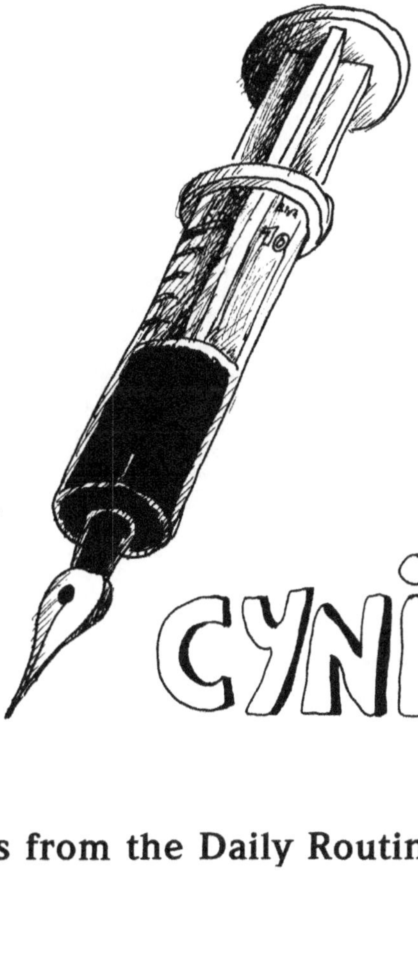

# MEDI CYNICAL

## Cartoons from the Daily Routine in Medicine

STEINKOPFF DARMSTADT

Prof. Dr. med. VOLKER LANGE
Schlosspark-Klinik
Abteilung Chirurgie
Heubnerweg 2
14059 Berlin, Germany

Title of the Original German Edition:
Mit schwarzem Strich. Cartoons aus dem medizinischen Alltag
Volker Lange, Berlin


ISBN 978-3-7985-1431-7 ISBN 978-3-642-57366-8 (eBook)
DOI 10.1007/978-3-642-57366-8

Cataloging-in-Publication Data applied for
A catalog record for this book is available from the Library of Congress.
Bibliographic information published by Die Deutsche Bibliothek
Die Deutsche Bibliothek lists this publication in the Deutsche Nationalbibliografie, detailed bibliographic data is available in the Internet at <http://dnb.ddb.de>.



http://www.steinkopff.springer.de


Originally published by Steinkopff-Verlag, Darmstadt in 2003



Translator: Seth Woodruff, Berlin, Germany

Production and Typesetting: druckerei justus kuch GmbH, Nürnberg
SPIN 10947432 105/7231-5 4 3 2 1 0 - Printed on acid-free paper.

# Foreword

Do cartoons that should speak to the observer themselves without using words require a foreword? Do Volker Lange's characteristic drawings, seen at least once by almost everyone involved with medicine, need description?

Does this book render more than a reason to laugh, more than a moment of 'aha'-experience, more than a fleeting instant of self-recognition? Do these cartoons convey more than ideas that may initially appear even absurd or bizarre?

Volker Lange has proven in previously published material that he knows how to disclose the perhaps intentionally overlooked parts of the medical profession. Here sideswipes against both physicians' vanity and the weight of the medical industry unmask much more than statements made by medical associations or auditing offices. Filled with warmhearted irony, but also biting sarcasm, Lange's cartoons testify to his sovereignability to analyze the business of medicine.

This book caricatures clinical medicine systematically. And almost every specialty – from general medicine to dentistry – serves as a target. The main focus, of course – no wonder considering the author's special field – involves the surgical disciplines, especially minimally invasive surgery and surgical endoscopy. In 'serious' medicine, Lange is proven expert in both.

Lange reveals the hidden dangers and pitfalls plaguing simple tasks in medicine such as measuring blood pressure and aural irrigation, but also those common to complex surgical procedures and the unfathomable depths of psychotherapy.

Within other cartoons, Lange details diverse horrors threatening the daily routine in surgery. Cartoons show fecal mist spraying from the rectoscope, the assistant's fingers being cut during skin incision, and the difficulties met by medullary nailing. Elsewhere in the book, the flexible endoscope becomes a snake, 'Nessie' swims in the disinfection basin, and Laokoon and sons fight against an endoscope. Seen from Lange's perspective, concepts such as the drawer phenomenon, an onychomycosis, and the appendix appear in unique, new light.

Lange's cartoons depict the grotesque, the mysterious, and the fantastic: patient and physician drowning in liquor during lumbal puncture, a patient actually coughing out his lungs, and a neurosurgeon, who finds emptiness when changing his patient's dressings, these are moments of enlightenment that free us from the bonds of a strictly scientific medicine fixed upon reality. Lange's book is a treasure chest of such surrealistic surprises.

With a few exceptions, Lange reveals his ideas using graphic expression only. Although his figures initially appear very much alike (like Loriot's and Mallet's bulbous-nosed characters), discrete differences in mimic reveal their very distinct personalities. Masterly, how Lange's masked surgeons come to speech!

Another unique feature of Lange's cartoons are the eyes of his conc-nosed characters. These are usually not drawn, and must be imagined behind the rimless glasses adorning each figure. Similar to the contrast in light and dark tones admired so much in Dutch paintings of the 17th century, clever hachures and etching lend depth to Lange's black-and-white scenes.

Despite catastrophic situations, Lange's characteristic faces lack great emotional expression. Indeed, only minor changes in body language allow us to suspect the pure horror facing each figure. Moreover, in each picture, an almost melancholic moment-in-time seems to contradict the highly dramatic situation illustrated. Exactly this cleverly composed contrast induces an almost unbearable emotional stress in the observer that subsides only by laughing.

Lange's illustrations are mostly original. Exceptions include historical references, associations, and quotations such as the 'skin decollement' by Serre and the 'exorcist' lurking outside the operating room. These borrowed excerpts complement Lange's cleverly placed novel ideas.

This cartoon collection prompts quick laughter, but also conveys the critical impressions of a modern physician confronted by a somewhat questionable medicine, one which most of us take for granted.

In addition to addressing various uncommon aspects of the medical profession (reanimation in the living room, emergency intervention at the site of an accident), Lange also caricatures several so-called medical 'advancements'. Using minimally invasive surgery as an example, the author draws a critical question mark behind modern medicine's dependence upon technology. High-tech used as a toy by the child in the surgeon, high-tech, replacing both handwork and artistry – these pictures invite us to reevaluate or belief in 'progress'.

Contemporary cartoon criticizing medicine follow many historical examples. William Hogarth, Gustave Doré, Honoré Daumier and others questioned, criticized, and denounced physicians and new therapies in a sharp and often aggressive manner. They portrayed physicians' inabilities and patients' fears using such pointed and caustic sarcasm, however, that the observer's laughter often remained stuck in his throat.

The aggressive sharpness common to medical cartoons of the 18th and 19th centuries has been replaced today by a vast number of mostly poor quality jokes about doctors. Indeed, the search for current medical humor equal to Eugen Roth's 'Wonder doctor' or to Wilhelm Busch's graphic and literary accomplishments is practically in vain. True humor –'the smiling acceptance of adversity', the 'nevertheless laughter' – is difficult to find in medicine, which remains inseparably connected to sickness and death, operation and complication, and the abyss of human existence. Examples of such humor, however, may include the Miraculix figure in 'Asterix', Dr. Zook, the doctor in Dick Brown's 'Hägar', and 'Peanuts' by Charles Schultz.

Lange's cartoons include elements derived from both perspectives, the caustic-cynical and the conciliatory-philosophical. The previously mentioned melancholic moment-in-time that seems to capture his figures may reflect an equilibrium found between these two perspectives, between 'aggressive' and 'resignative smiling' reactions to adversity.

In summary, this medical-satirical picture book deserves to be a great success. The cartoons should serve many readers – especially those involved with surgery – as a source of 'recreation of the mind', particularly during difficult times. In addition, some observers may experience a certain degree of self-recognition. Colleagues may suddenly see both themselves and their profession in an amusing, sometimes critical, new light. And so the timeless ΓΝΩΘΙ ΣΑΥΤΟΝ – the 'cognosce te ipsum' of the oracle of Delphi – imparts its healing power today through the medical cartoon.

Tübingen,
Summer 2003

Prof. Dr. K.E. Grund
Surgical Endoscopy
University Hospital
72076 Tübingen

# PREFACE

The less text found between two book covers, the more necessary the preface becomes. A photo album submitted without an imposing, clarifying introduction – impossible! A compilation of paintings presented without analytical classification or reference to art history – totally unthinkable! And a cartoon collection? There's a dilemma. Basically, the author of the following book simply decided to express himself without using text. Rarely, because of poor writing ability, more often, due to a wise self-recognition that he should not write, and sometimes, after reaching a kind of philosophical state-of-mind, because he did not want to write. That explains just about everything. Because the publisher, expecting more of an introduction, planned more room here, however, I am compelled to share a few details on the making of this book with my reader. These details are of course absolutely unnecessary for understanding or enjoying the cartoons contained in this book.

My admired, but feared high school German teacher labelled the cartoons that I published in the student magazine 'lesser art'. That stigmatized my artistic efforts, and I decided, much to my parents' pleasure, to pursue a 'respectable' profession. I never did, however, entirely give up drawing. And when I began working as a physician, this hobby received a dynamic boost. Unbelievable what patients presented their doctors, and what doctors offered their patients! And then, all the wonderful instruments used to carry out diverse diagnostic tests and amazing methods of treatment! In short, a treasure chest of motifs materialized for the cartoonist, and my limited collection of cartoons gradually began to grow.

Still a resident, I published several cartoons on anesthesiology in the 'Deutsche Ärzteblatt' (1975), where they found warm approval. That was the beginning of sporadic publishing of other cartoons in various medical journals. A book on proctology followed. I put together a book highlighting the medical meeting, and created enough cartoons to make ten calendars. Thanks here once again to Mr. Gerd Rupp for bringing out the last eight. During numerous medical meetings, I have since seen many of the cartoons taken from these calendars presented as slides intended to liven up a presentation. There I sat quite satisfied in the audience...

Clinical medicine is above all empirical. As a result, the known begins to repeat itself after decades of work. Indeed, experience transforms once unfamiliar, strange land into a well-known home. Surprises become less frequent and inspiration for the cartoonist fades. This is especially true for the cartoonist who enjoys expressing his ideas solely through sketches, and not with the help of text placed in a speech bubble.

It was therefore high-time to come to an end, to finish this collection of cartoons, in order to direct my attention to new frontiers. While assessing the cartoons, I discovered that many drawn long ago no longer passed my own censorship. A few were revised, and a few were left unchanged, especially when reality had caught up with my fantasy. Examples of the latter include using a zipper to close a laparotomy and employing a robotic arm in minimally invasive surgery.

An assortment of cartoons has now been printed which the long-time friend, and those waiting for the new calendar, should recognize well. Everyone else will just have to take a look. That was also the view of Dr. G. Volkert, Steinkopff Verlag, whose enthusiasm and support helped create this book.

Berlin, Summer 2003 — Volker Lange

# GENERAL MEDICINE

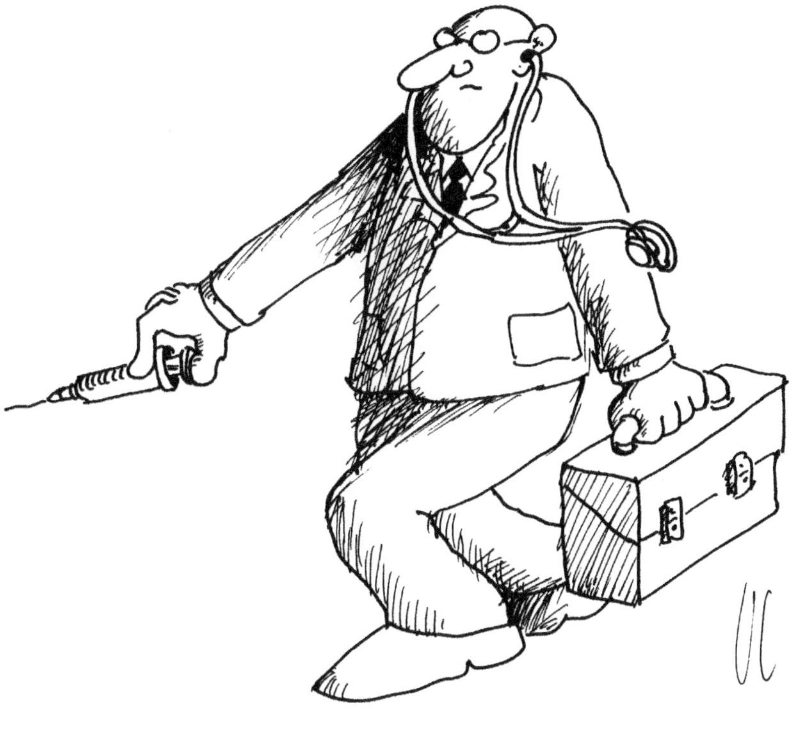

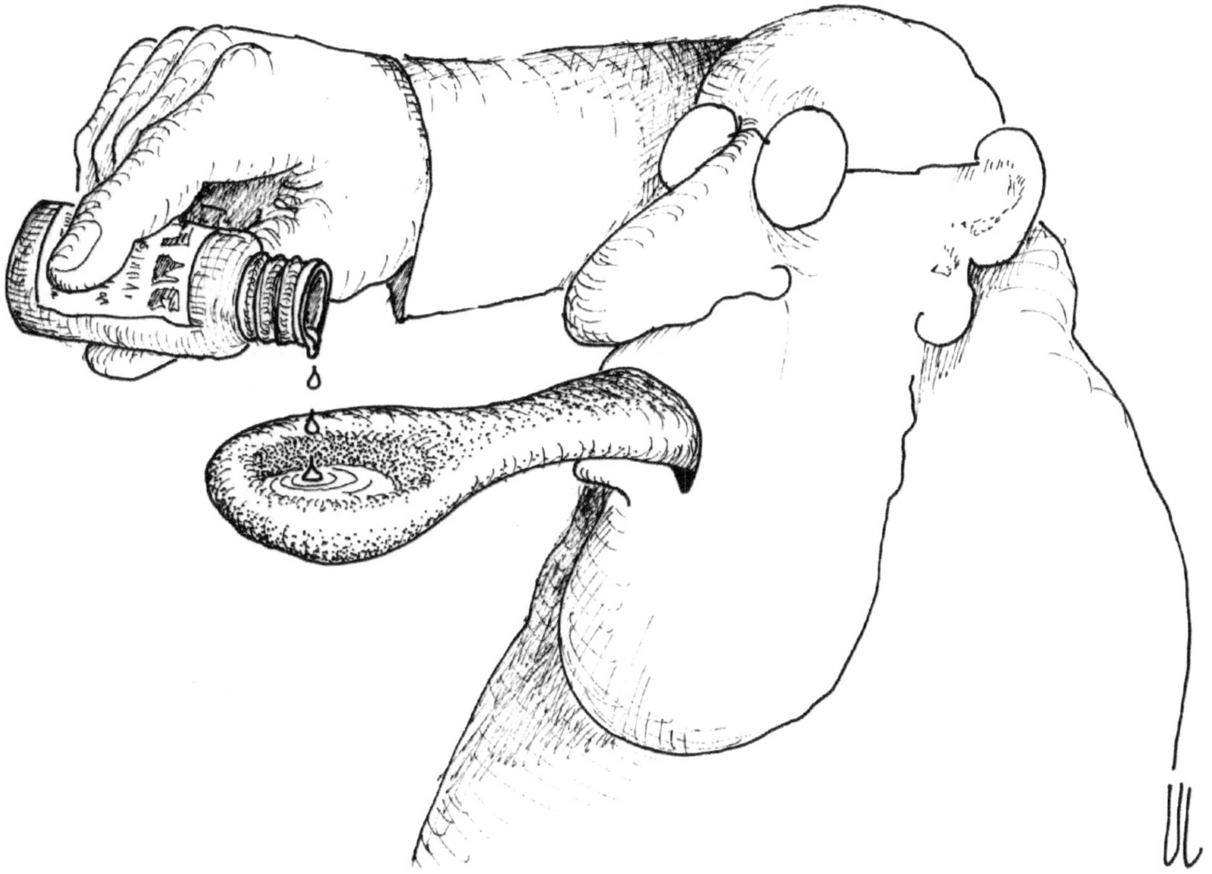

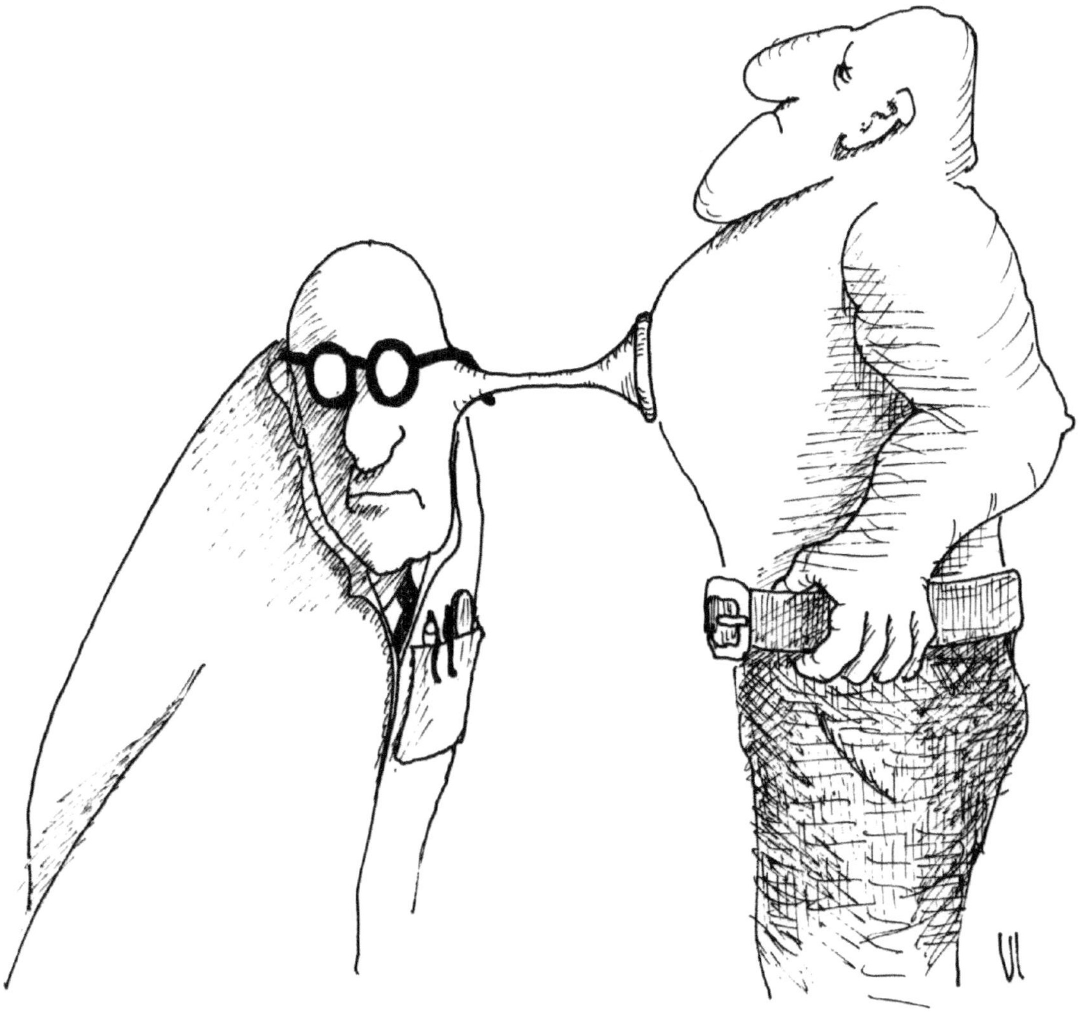

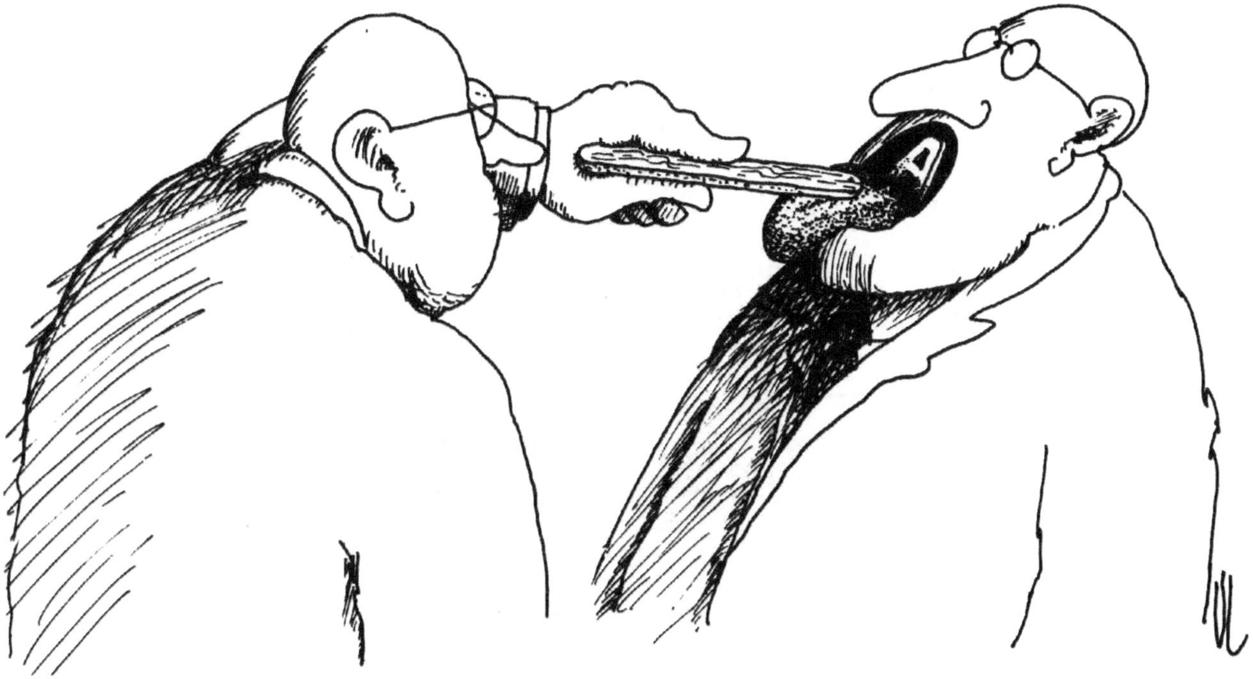

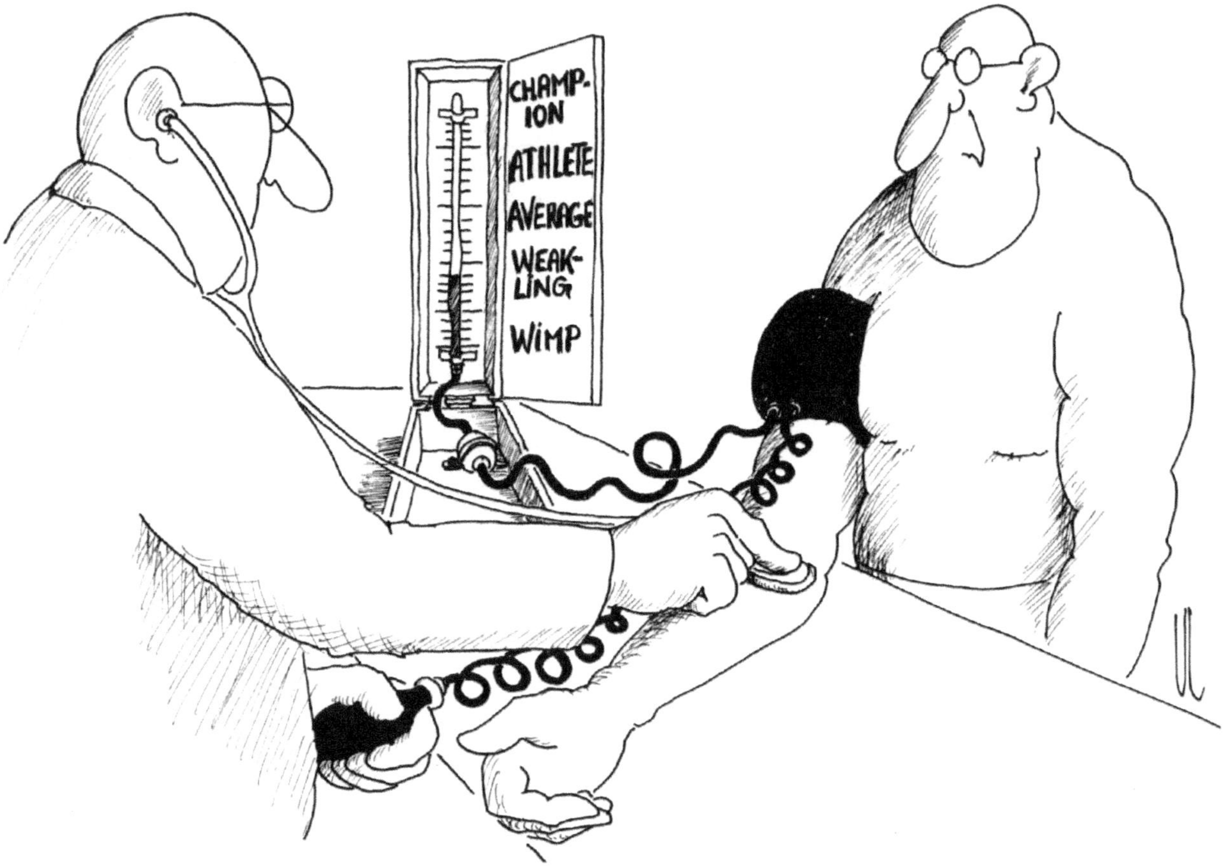
CHAMP-ION
ATHLETE
AVERAGE
WEAK-LING
WIMP

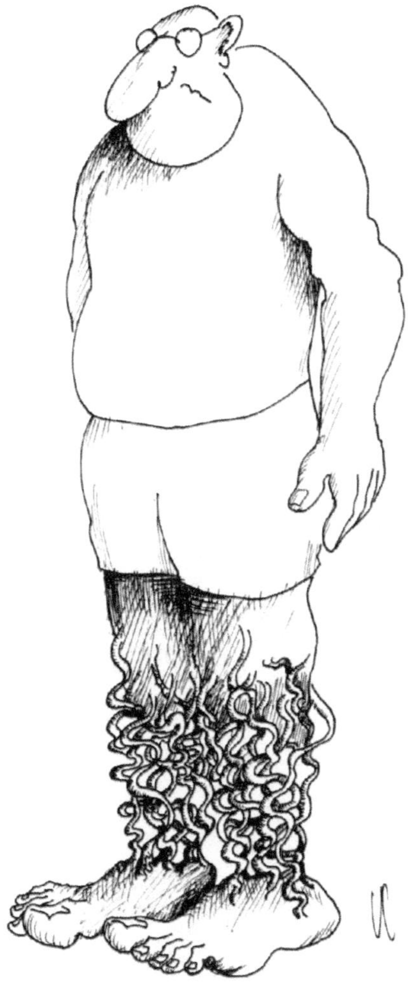

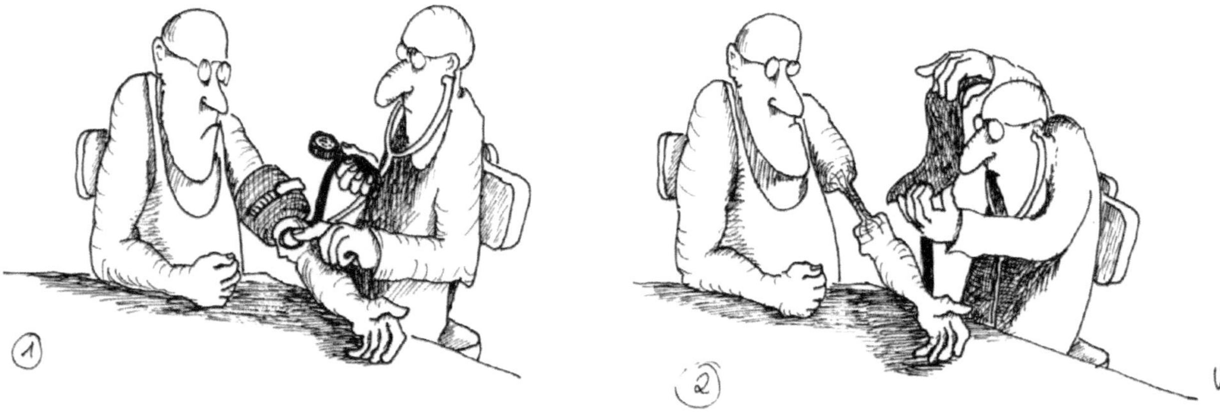
1
2

# ANESTHESIOLOGY

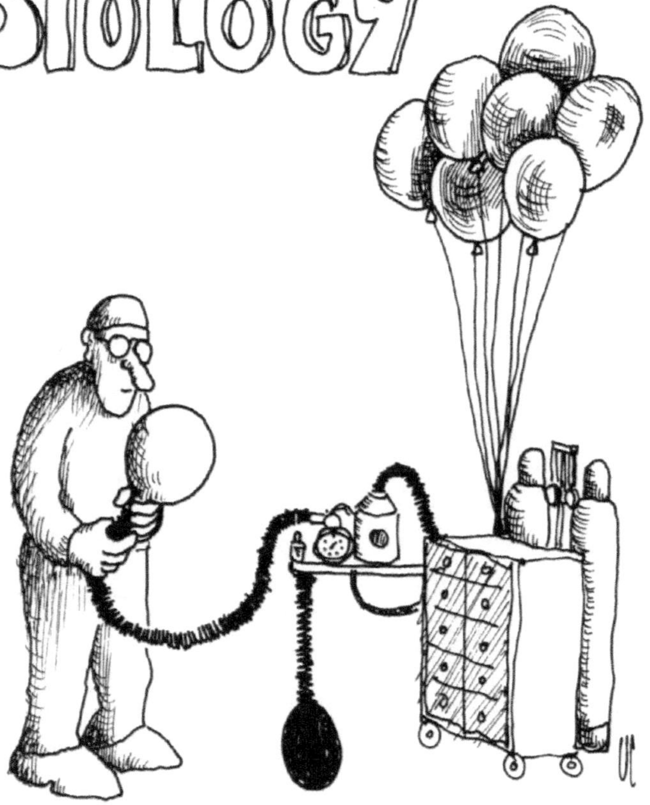

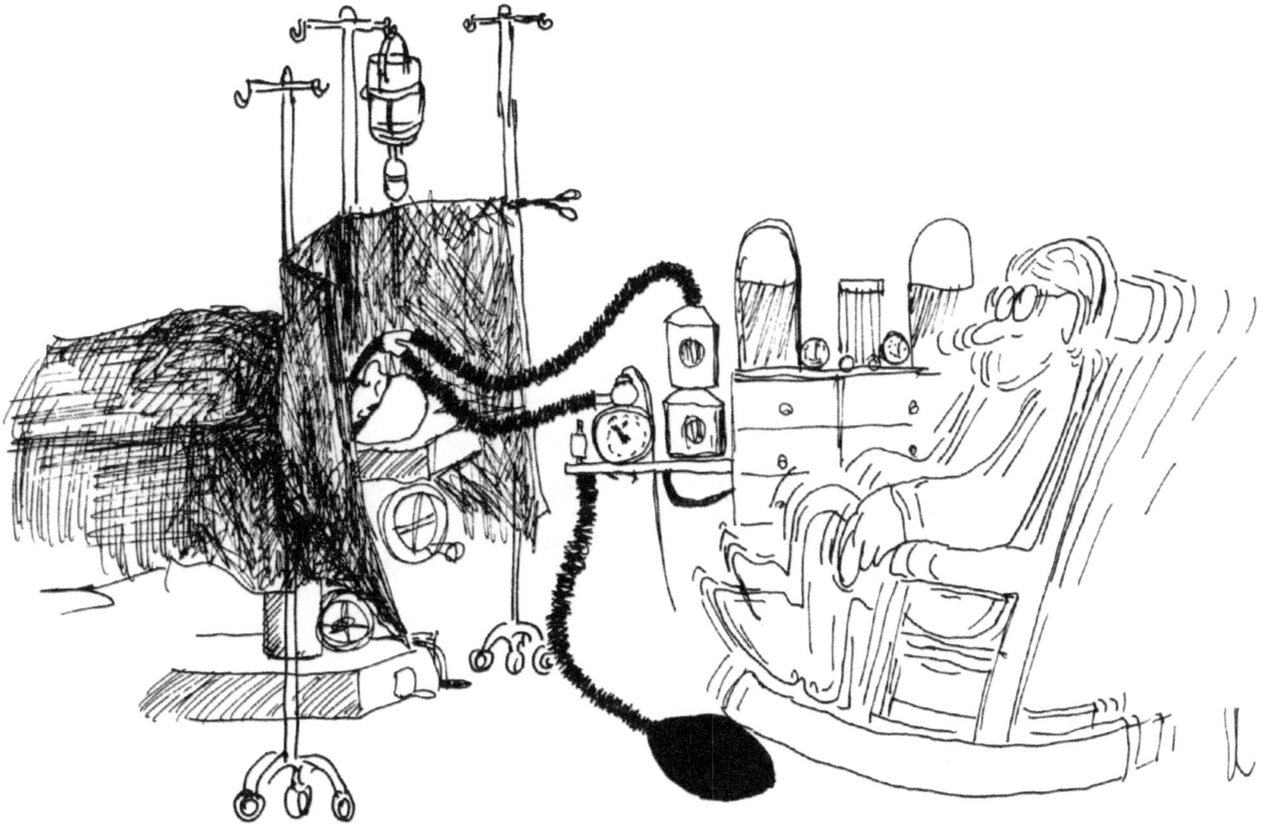

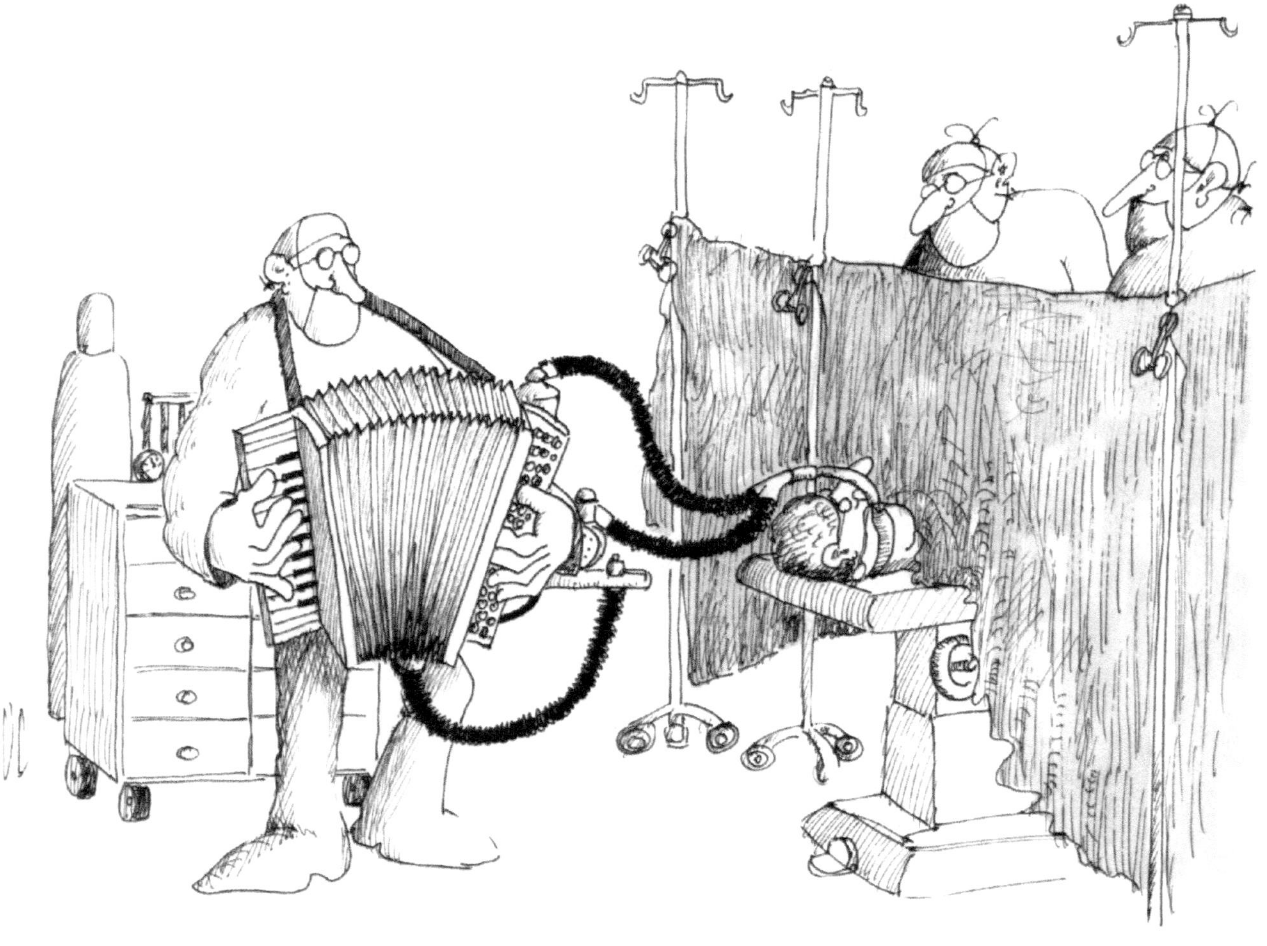

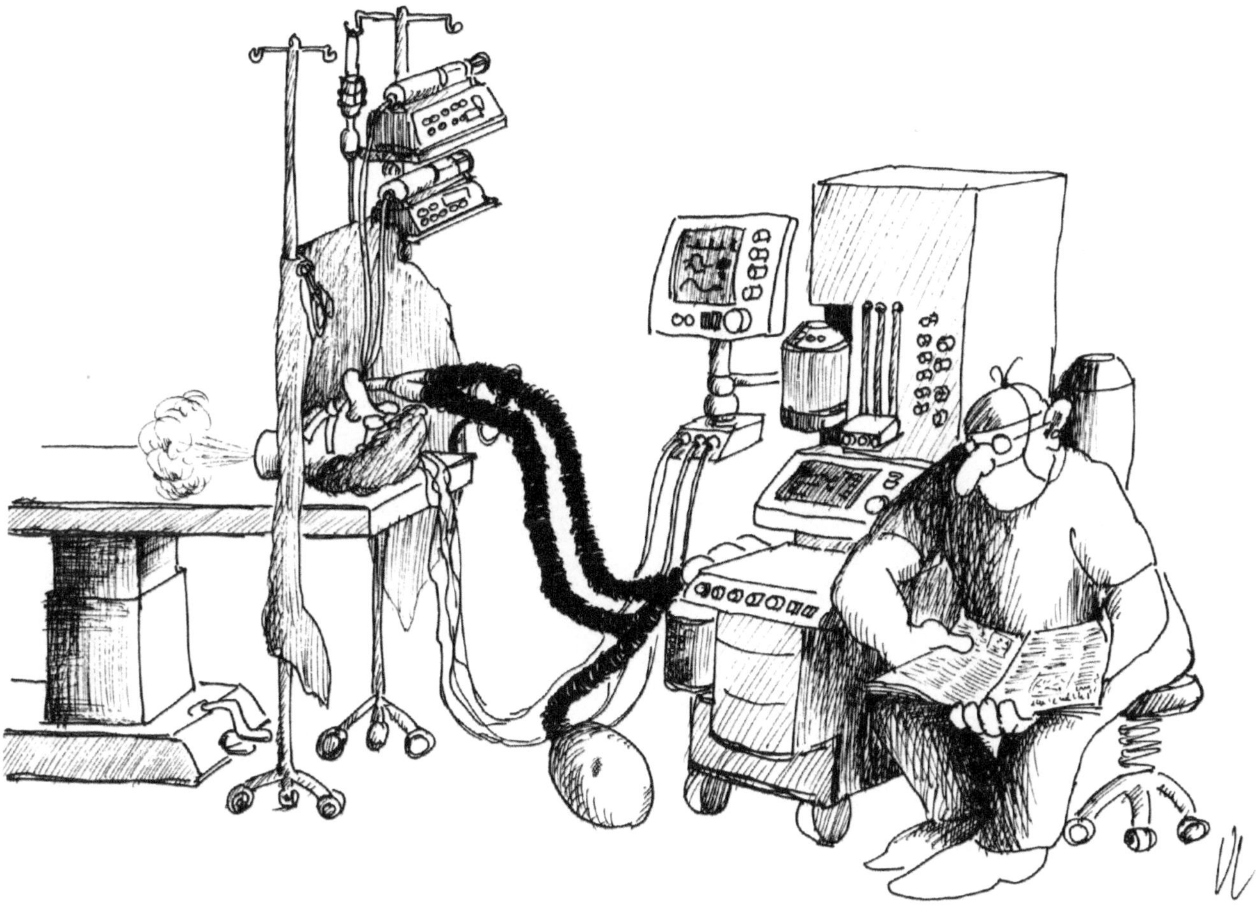

# SURGERY

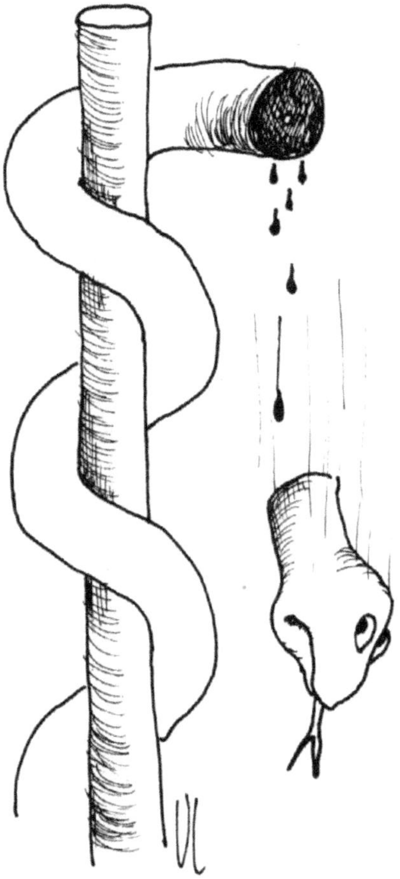

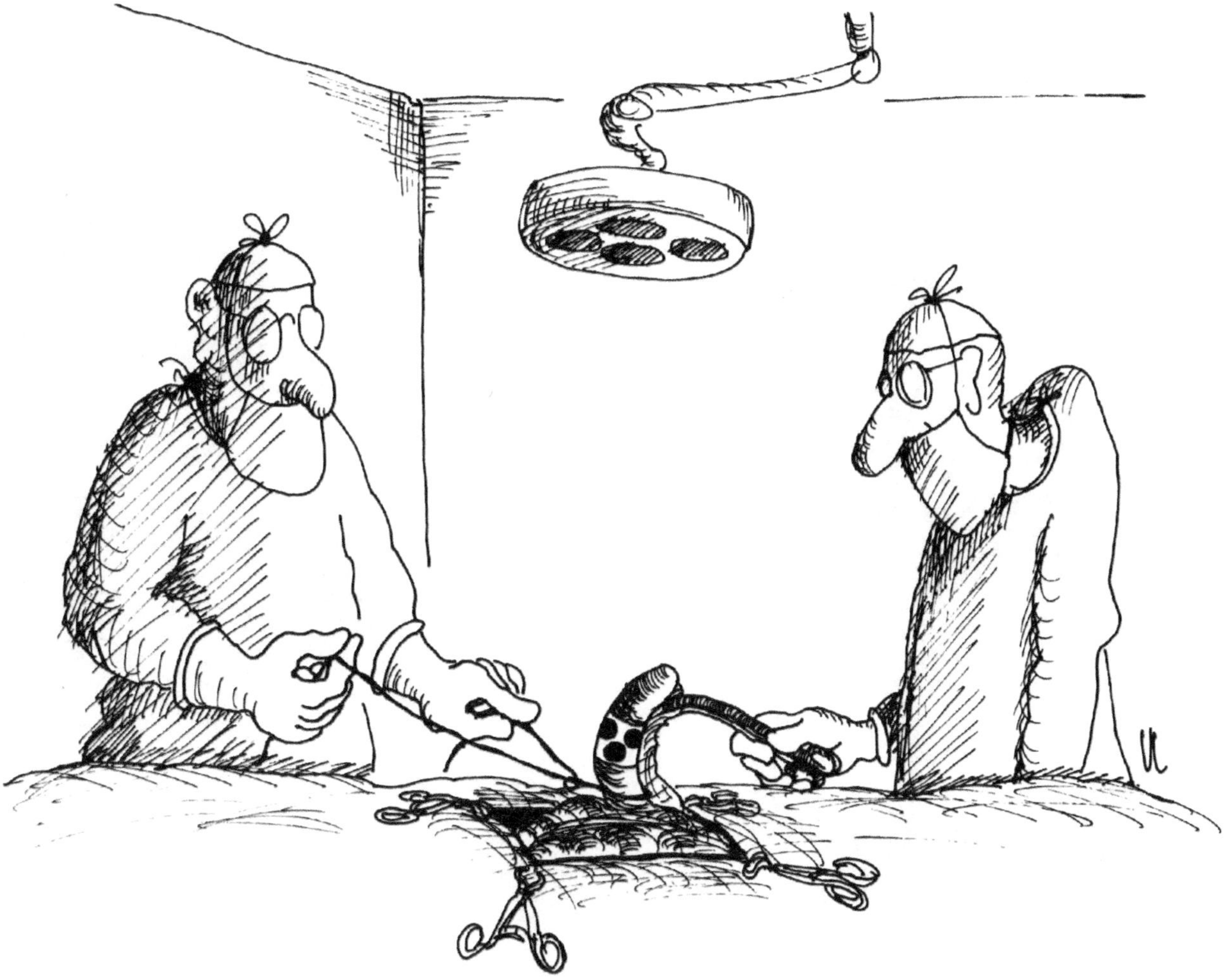

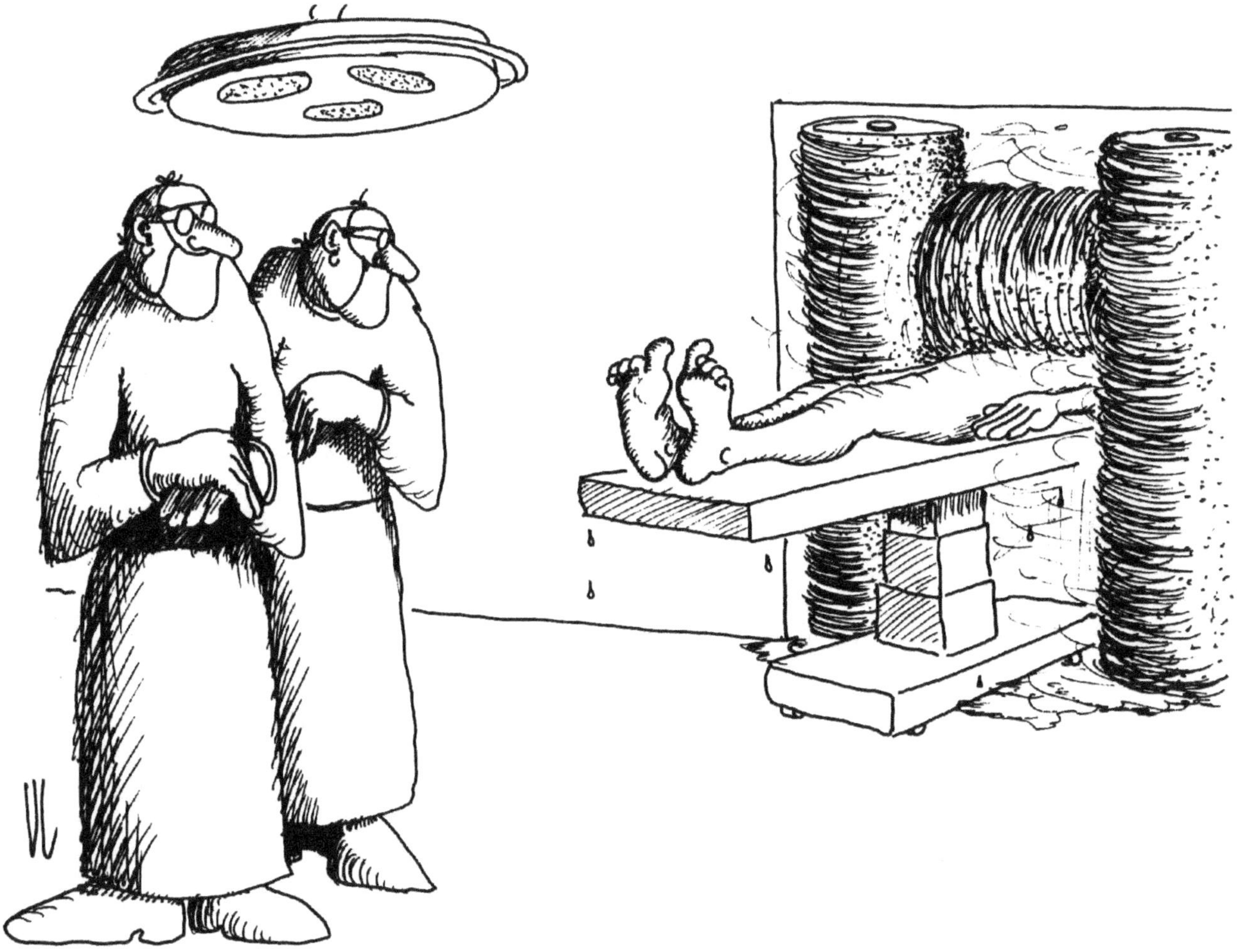

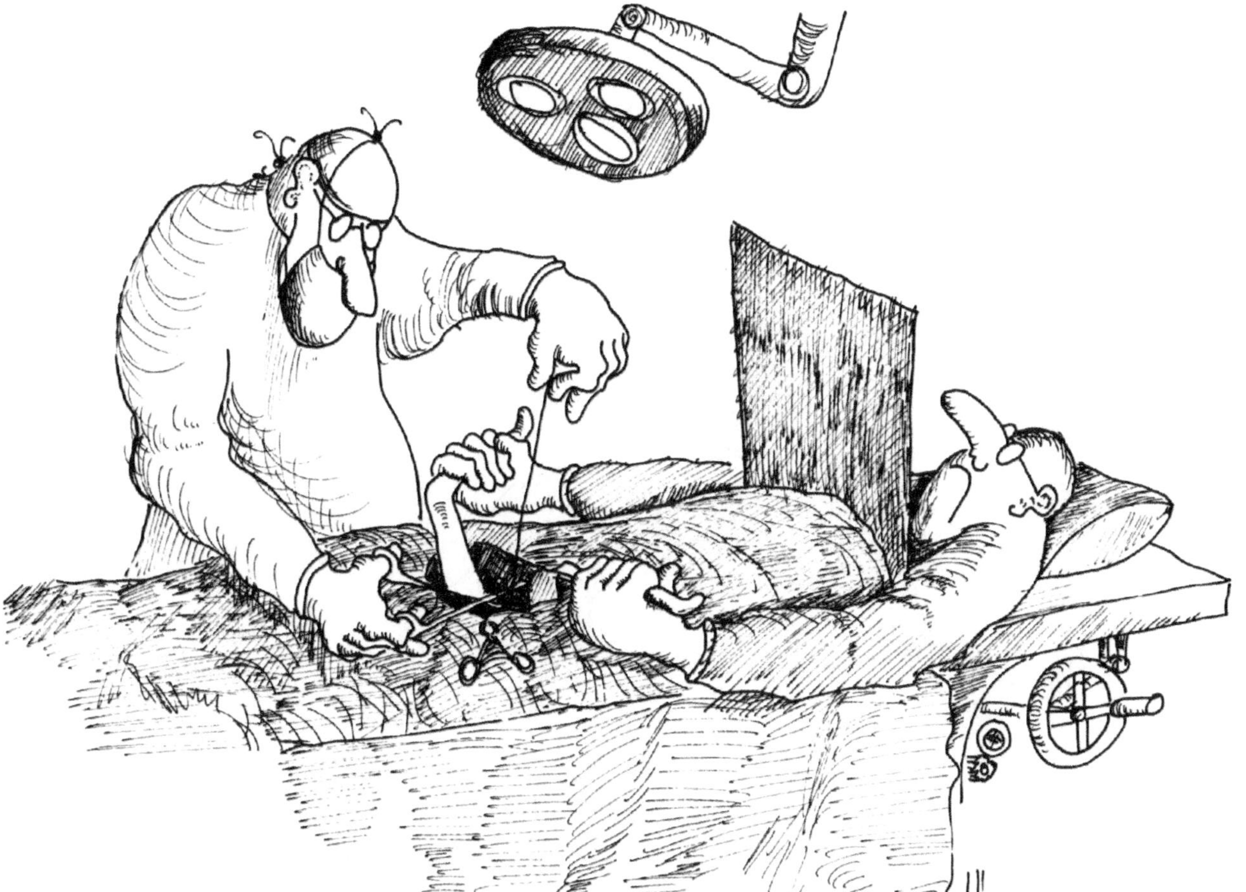

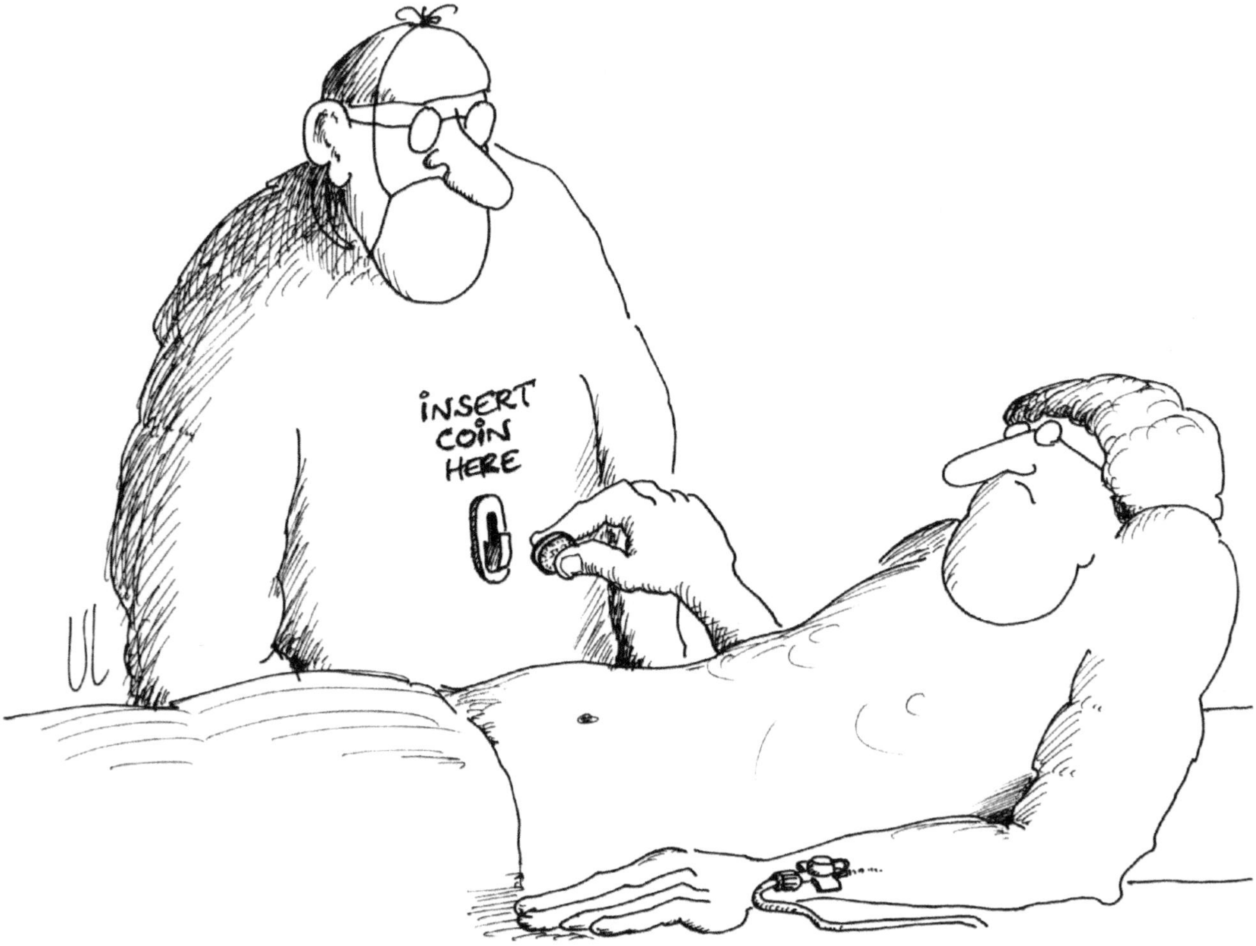
INSERT
COIN
HERE

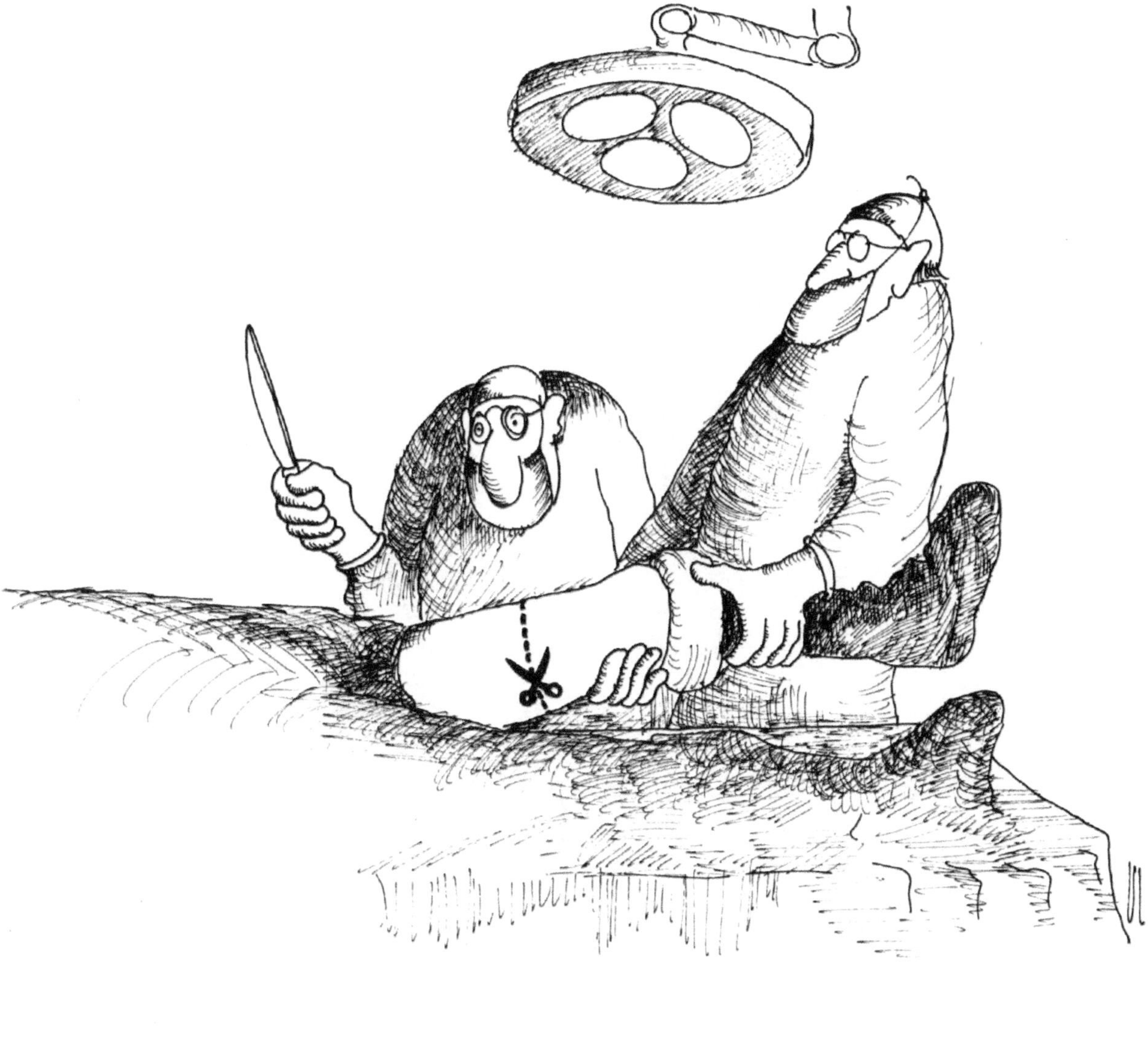

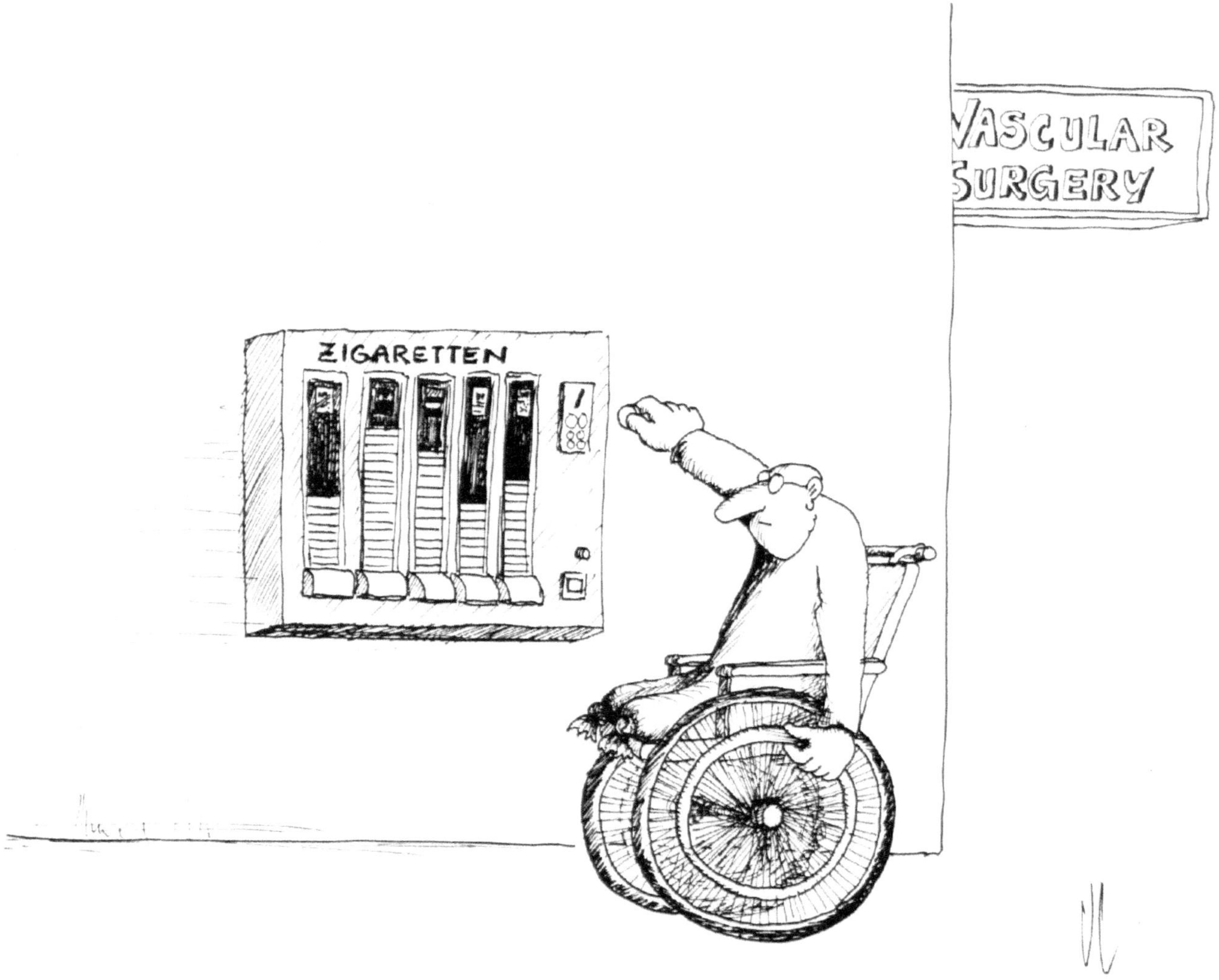
ZIGARETTEN
VASCULAR SURGERY

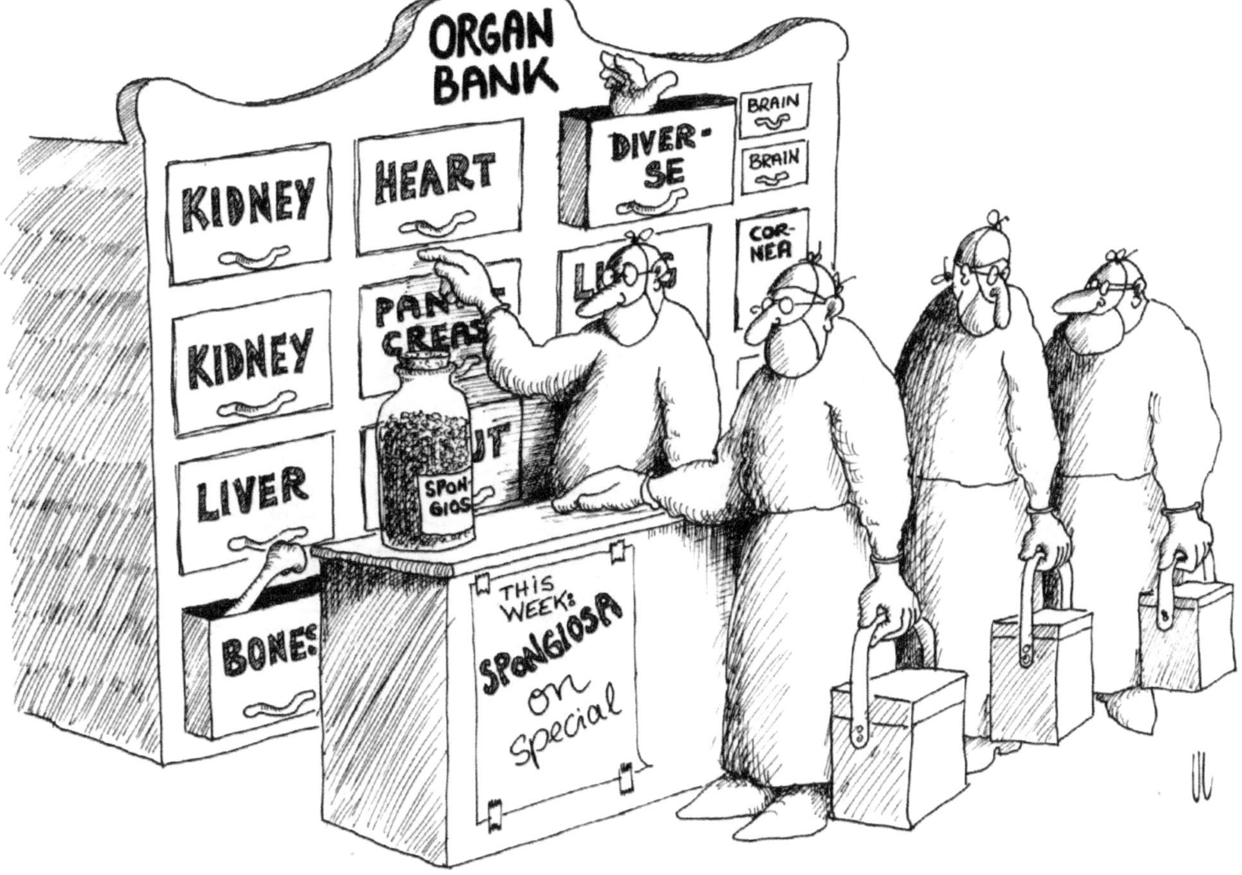
ORGAN
BANK
KIDNEY
HEART
DIVER-
SE
BRAIN
BRAIN
COR-
NEA
KIDNEY
LIVER
SPON-
GIOS
THIS
WEEK:
SPONGIOSA
on
special

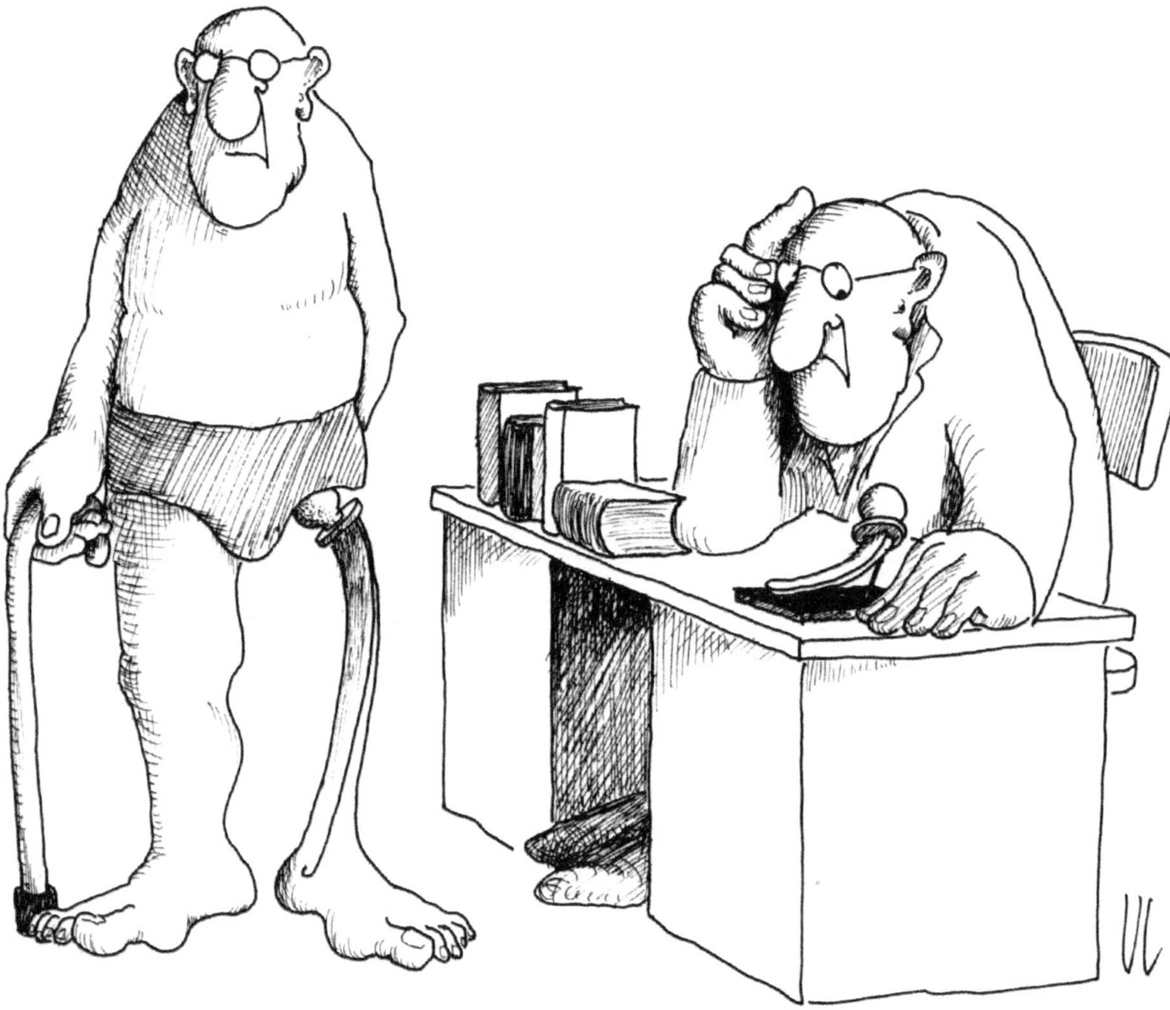

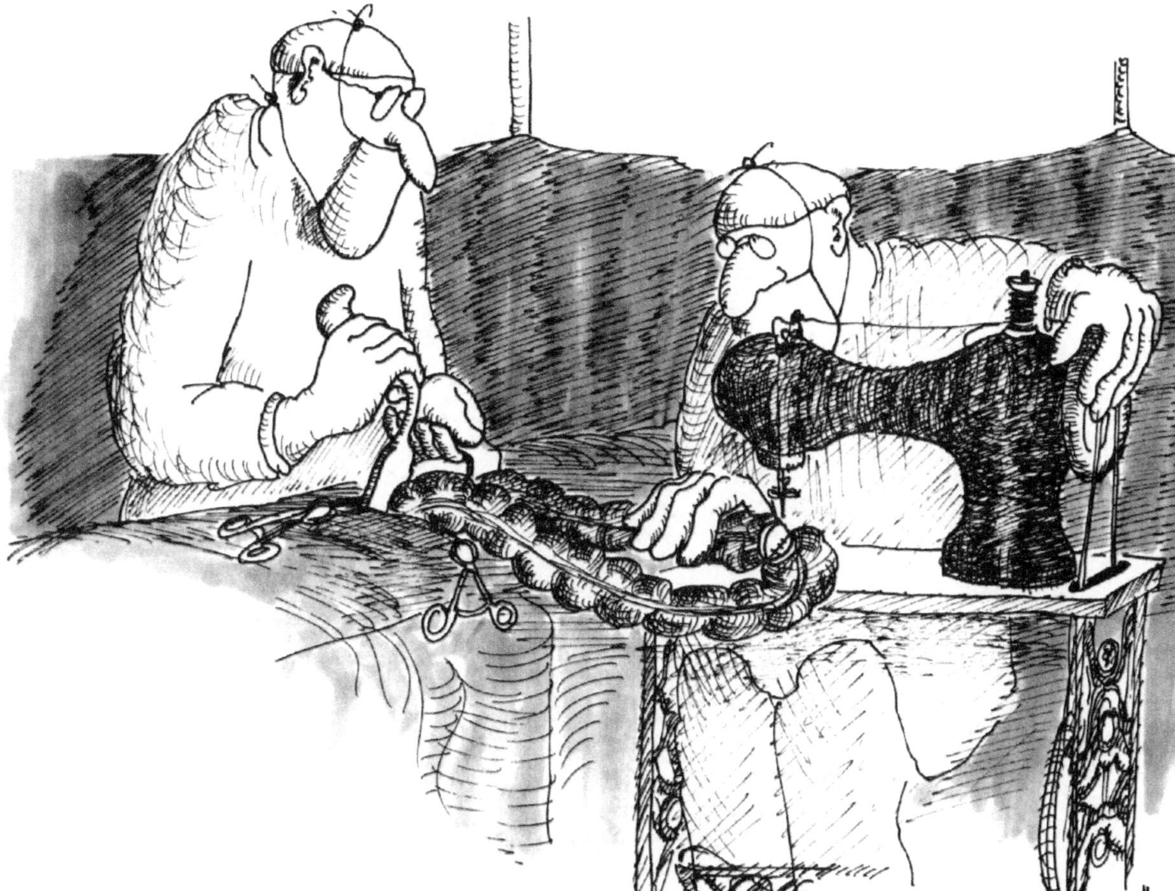

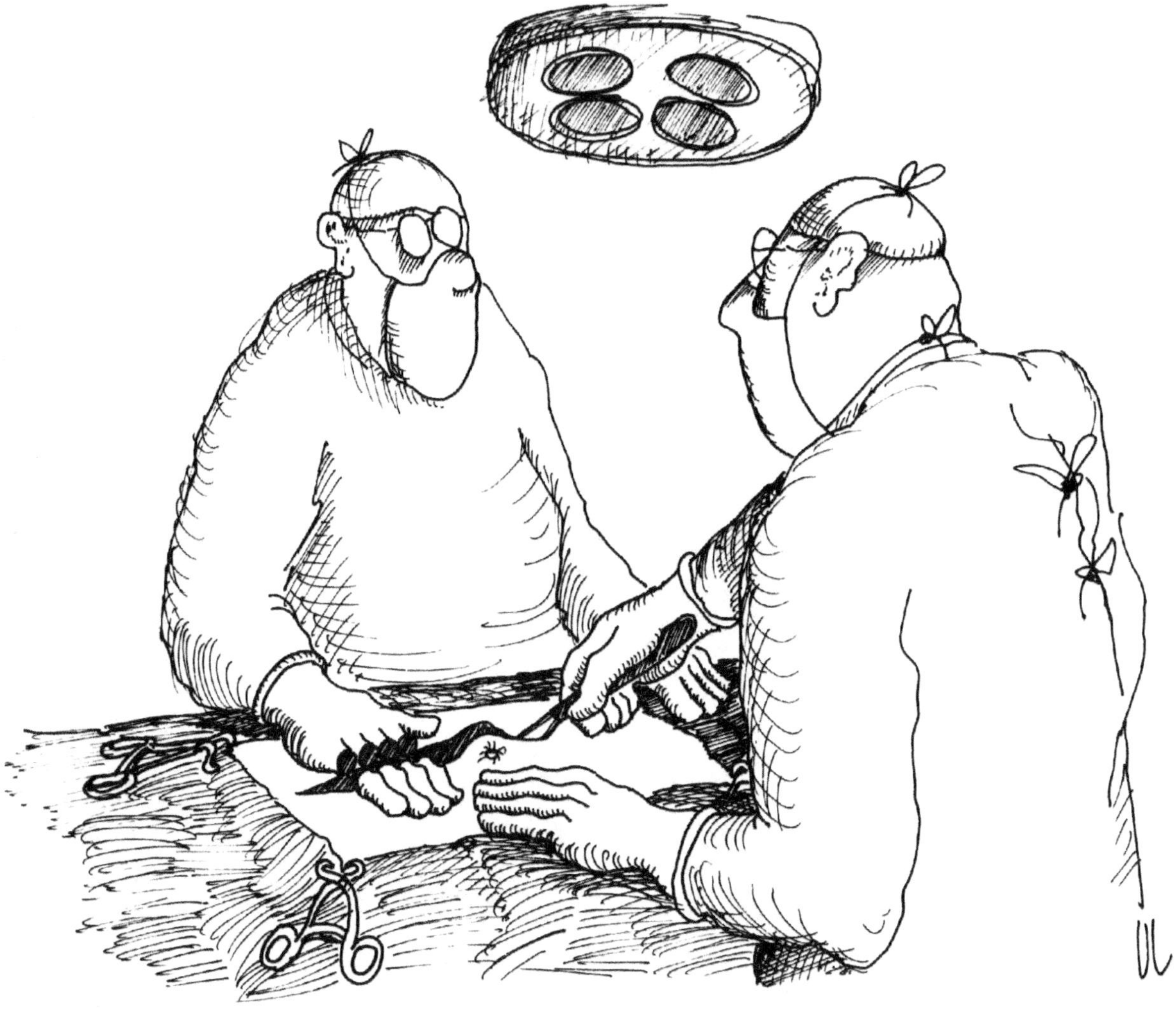

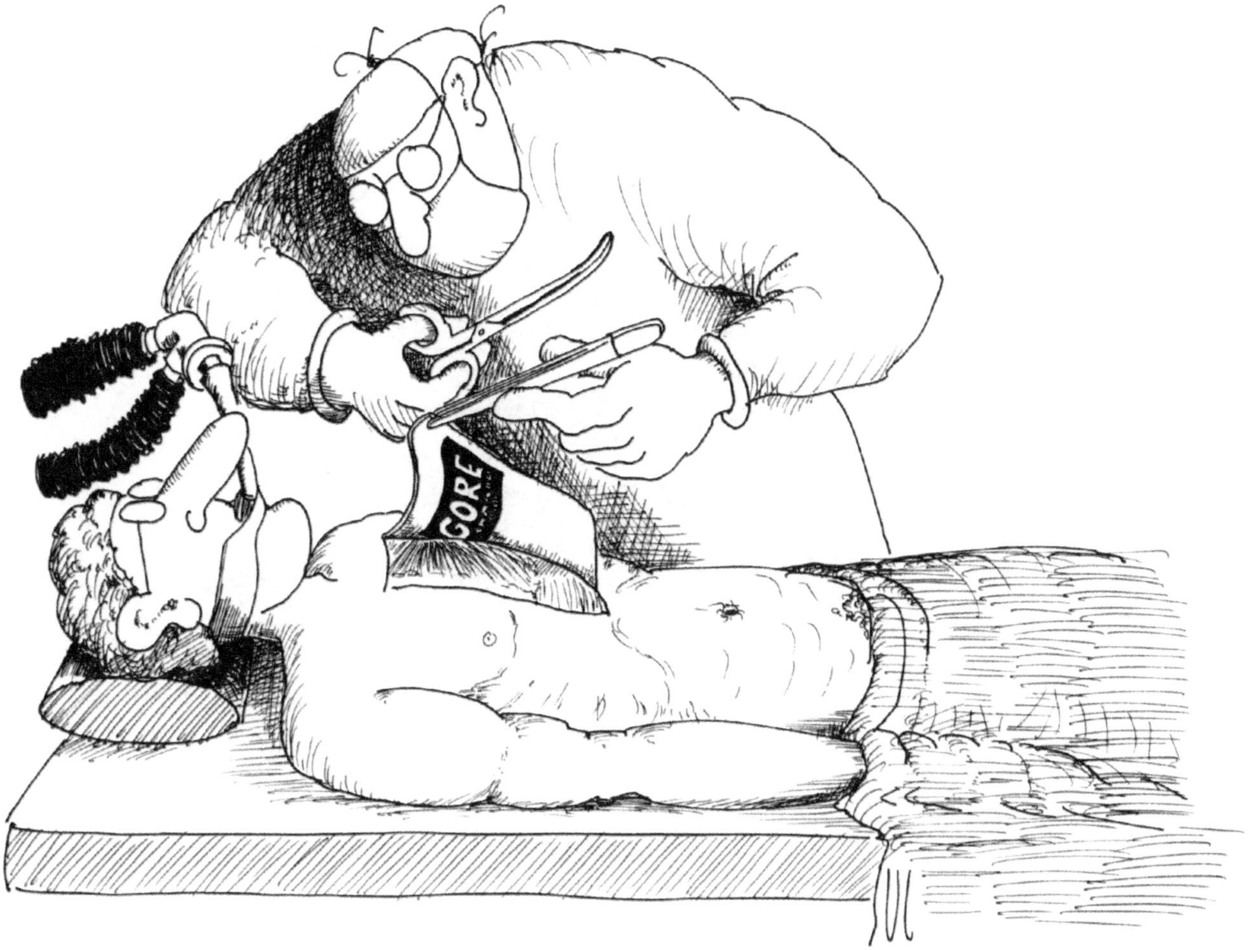
GORE

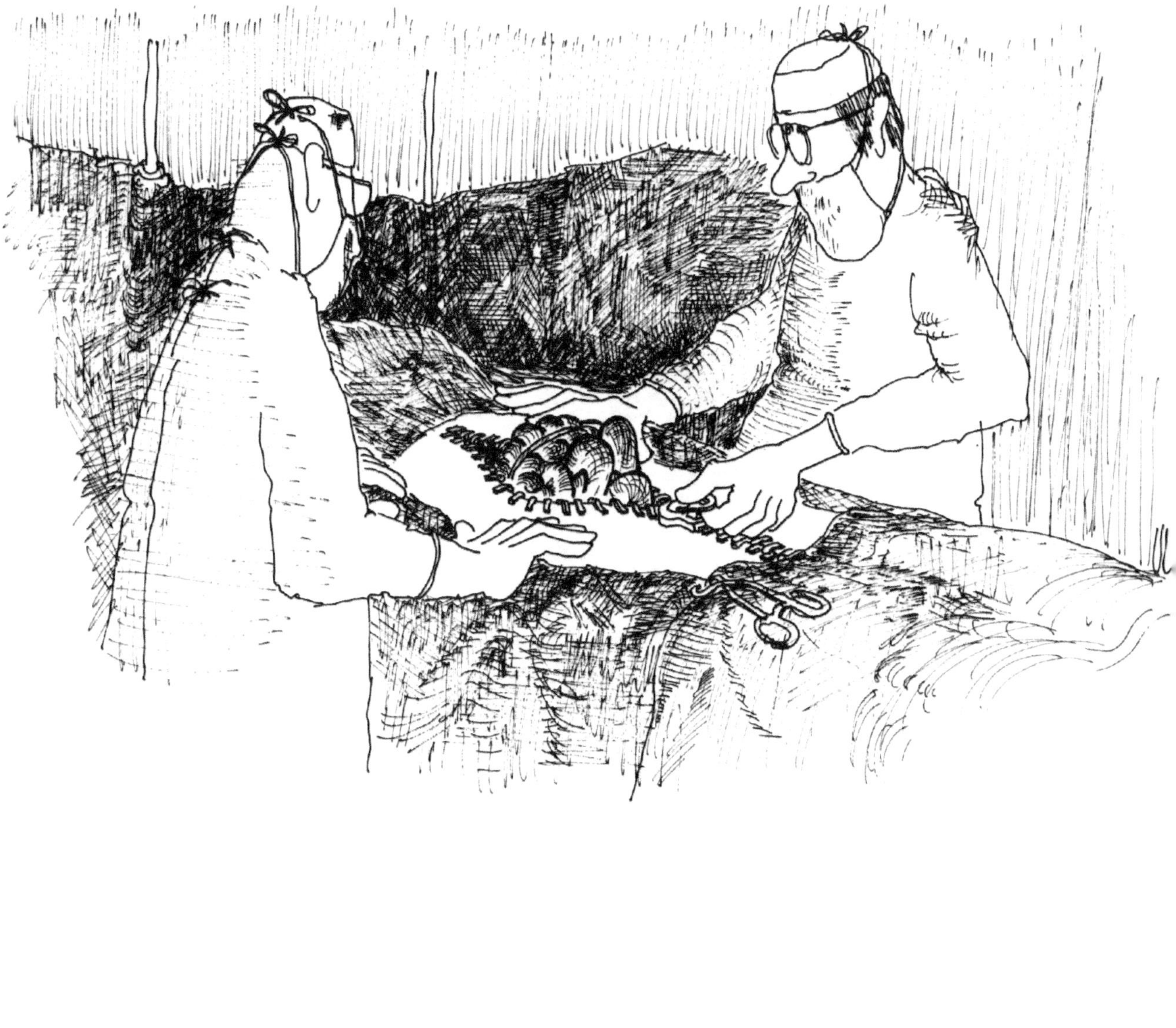

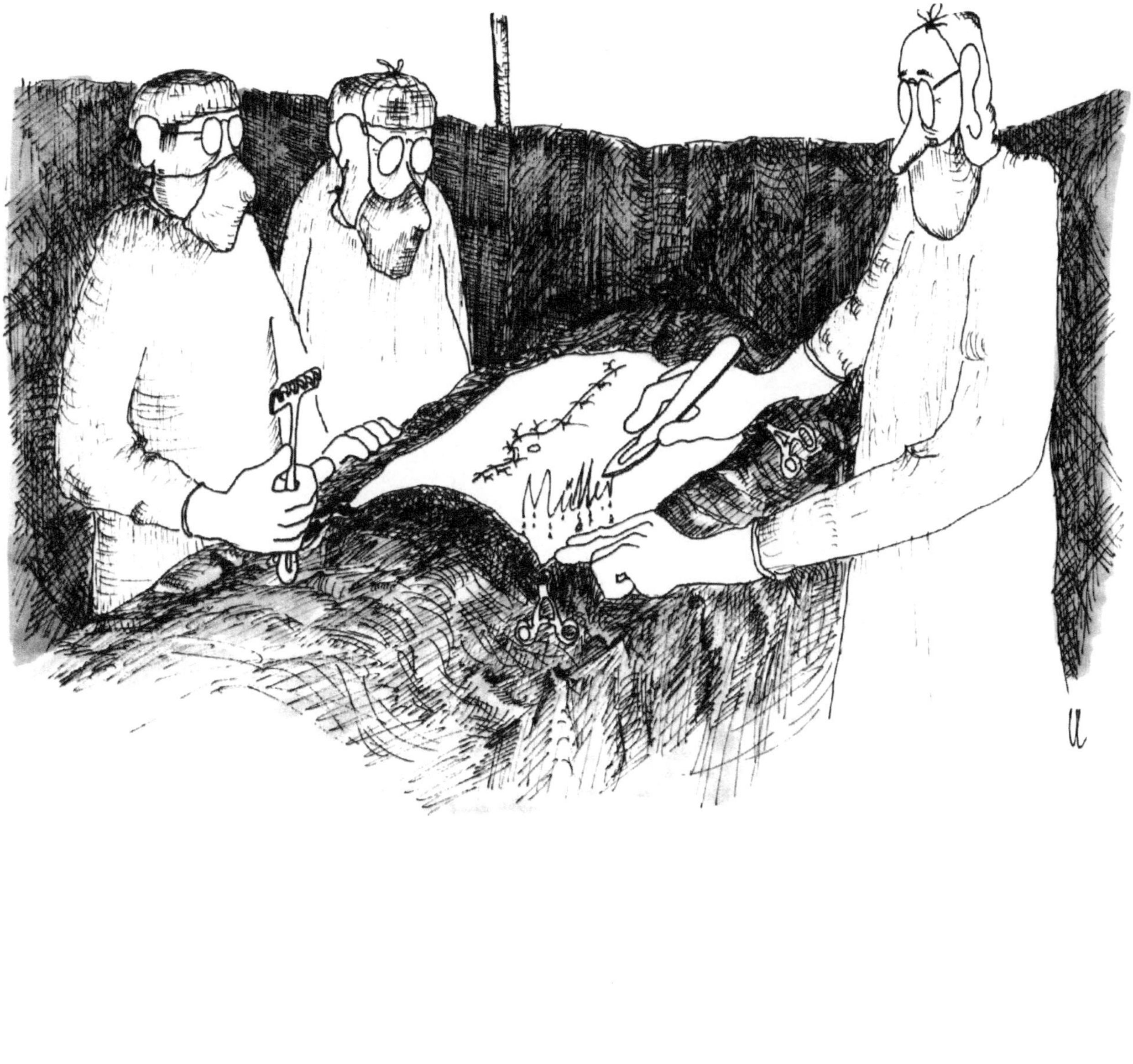
Müller

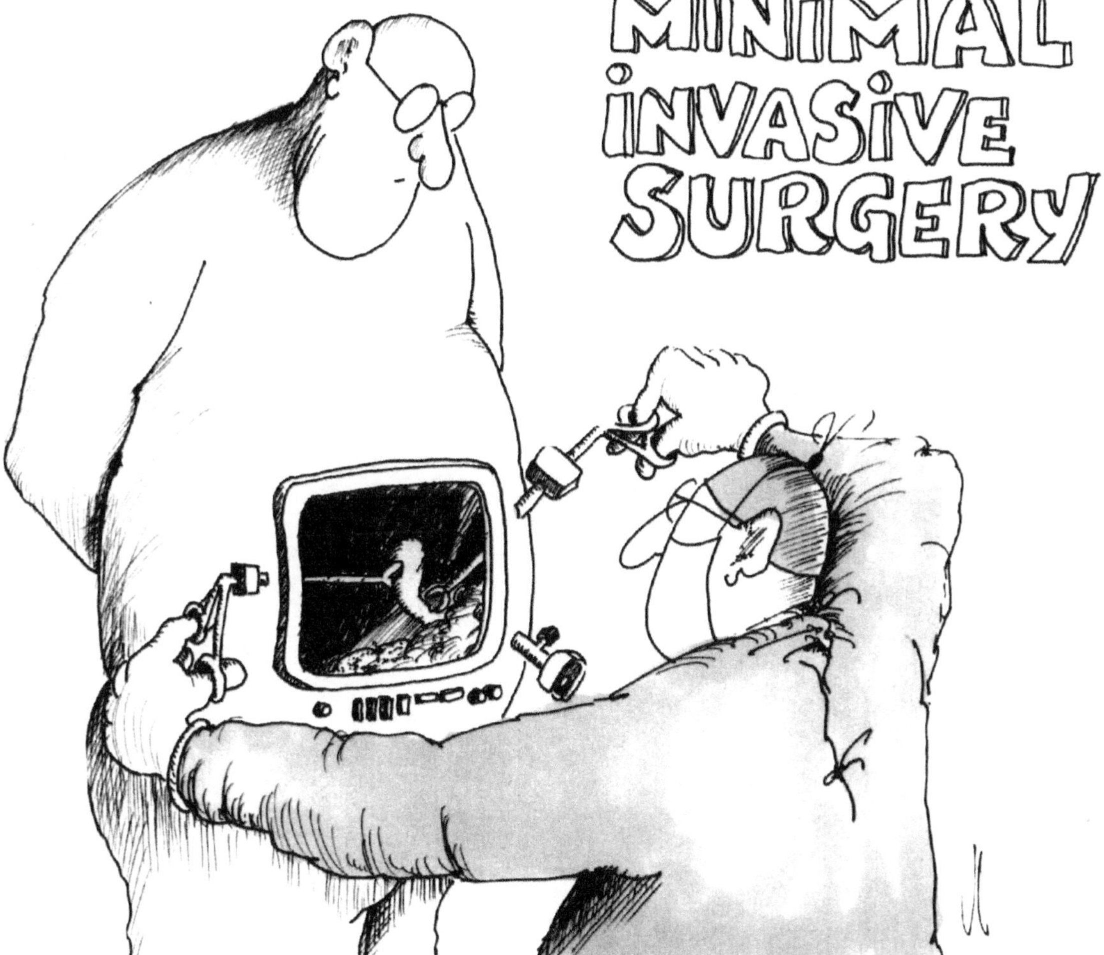
MINIMAL
INVASIVE
SURGERY

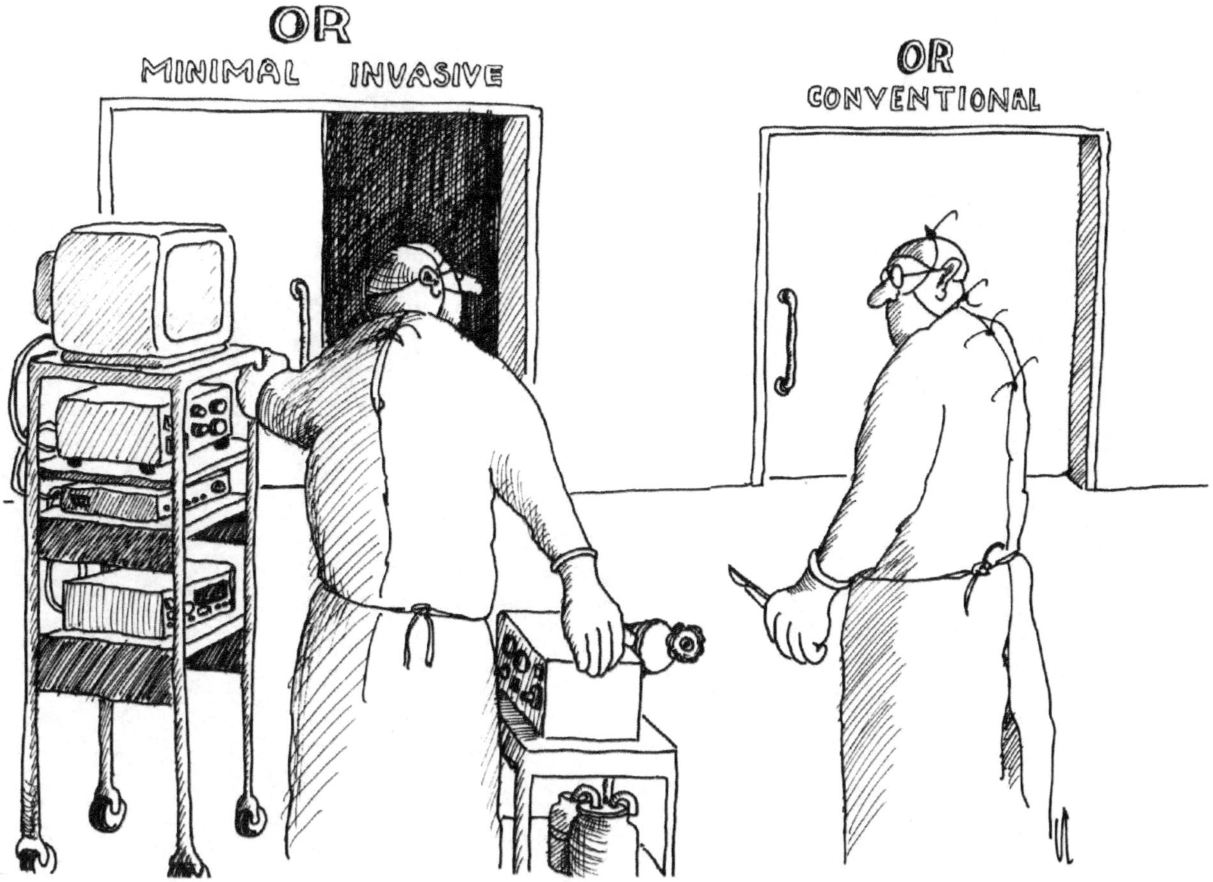
OR
MINIMAL INVASIVE
OR
CONVENTIONAL

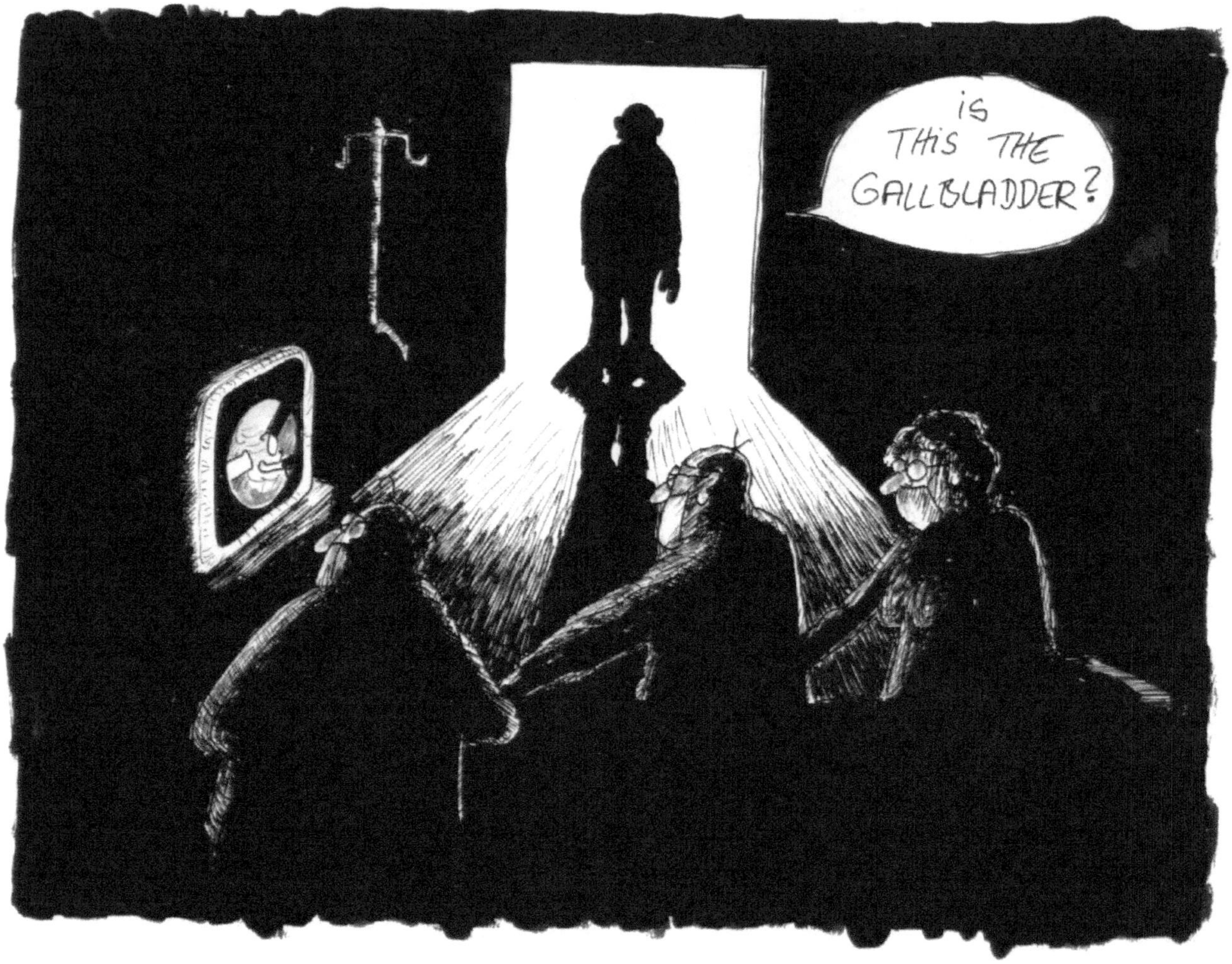
is THIS THE GALLBLADDER?

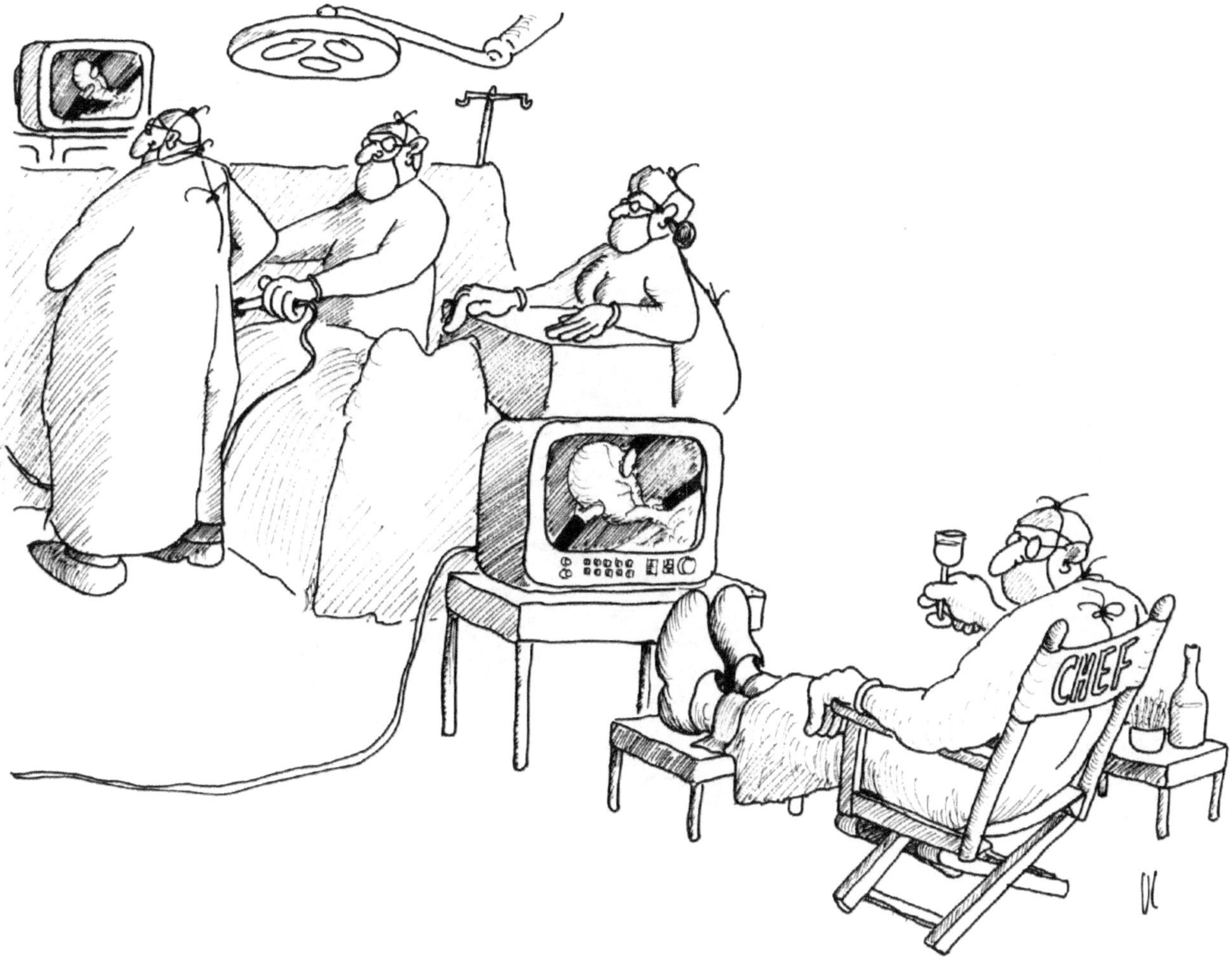
CHEF

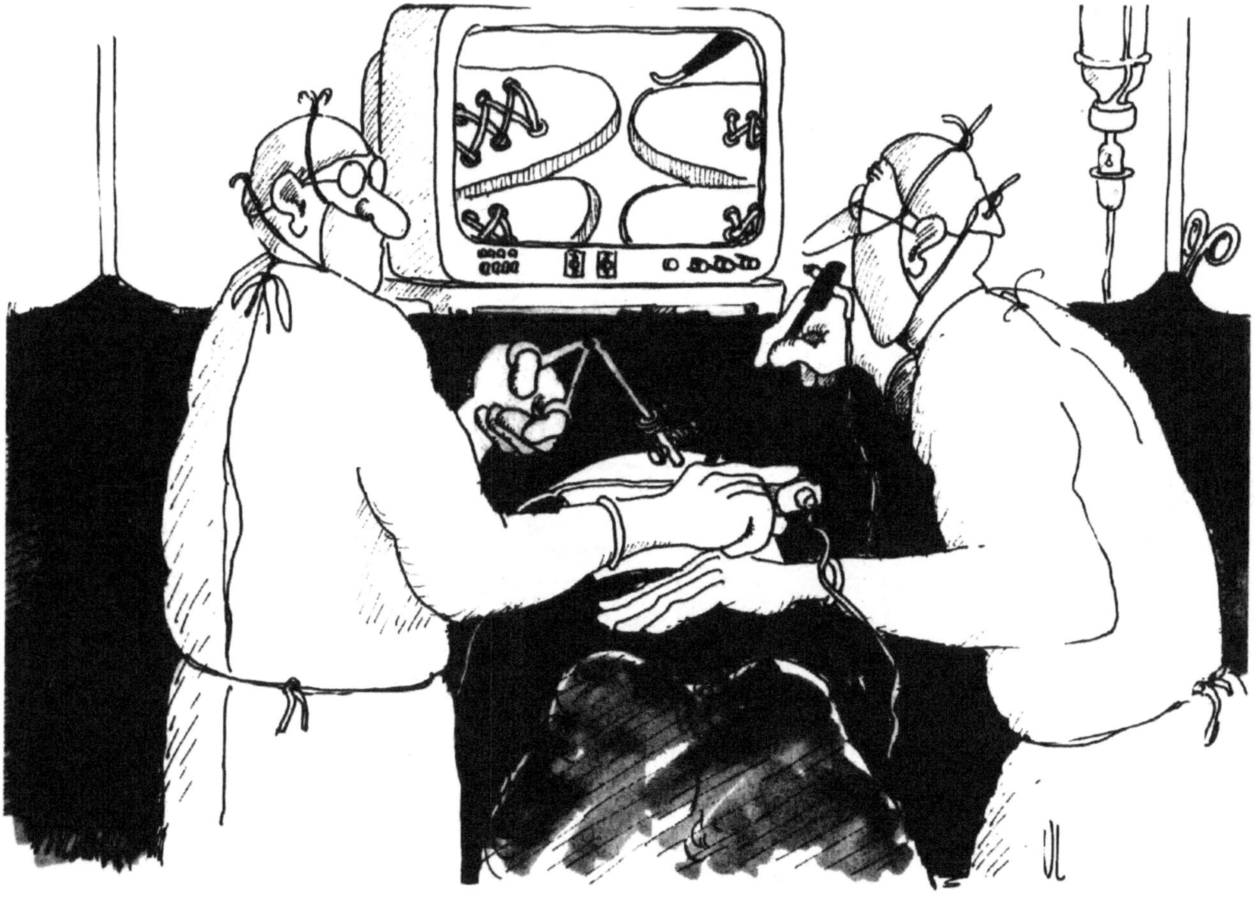

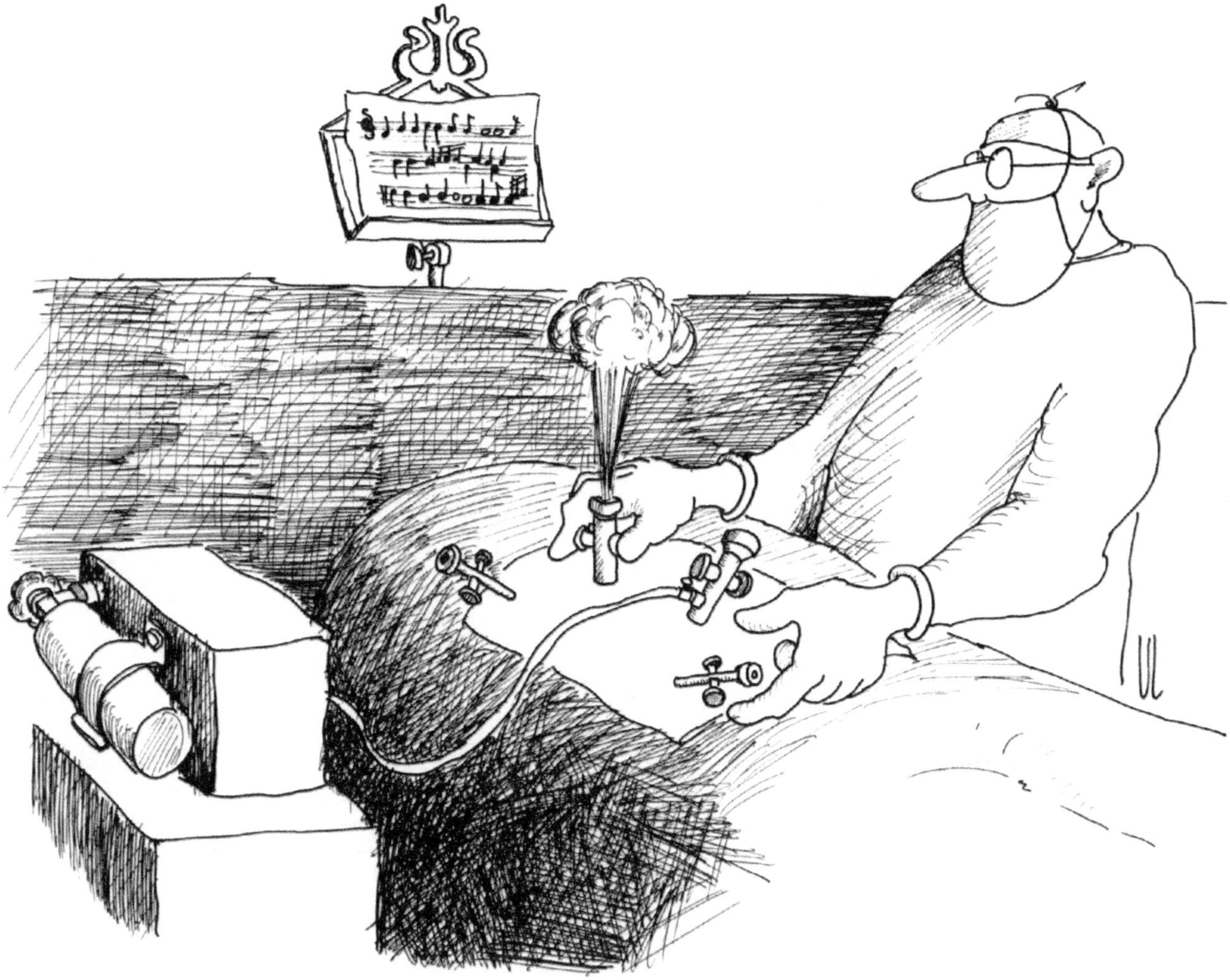

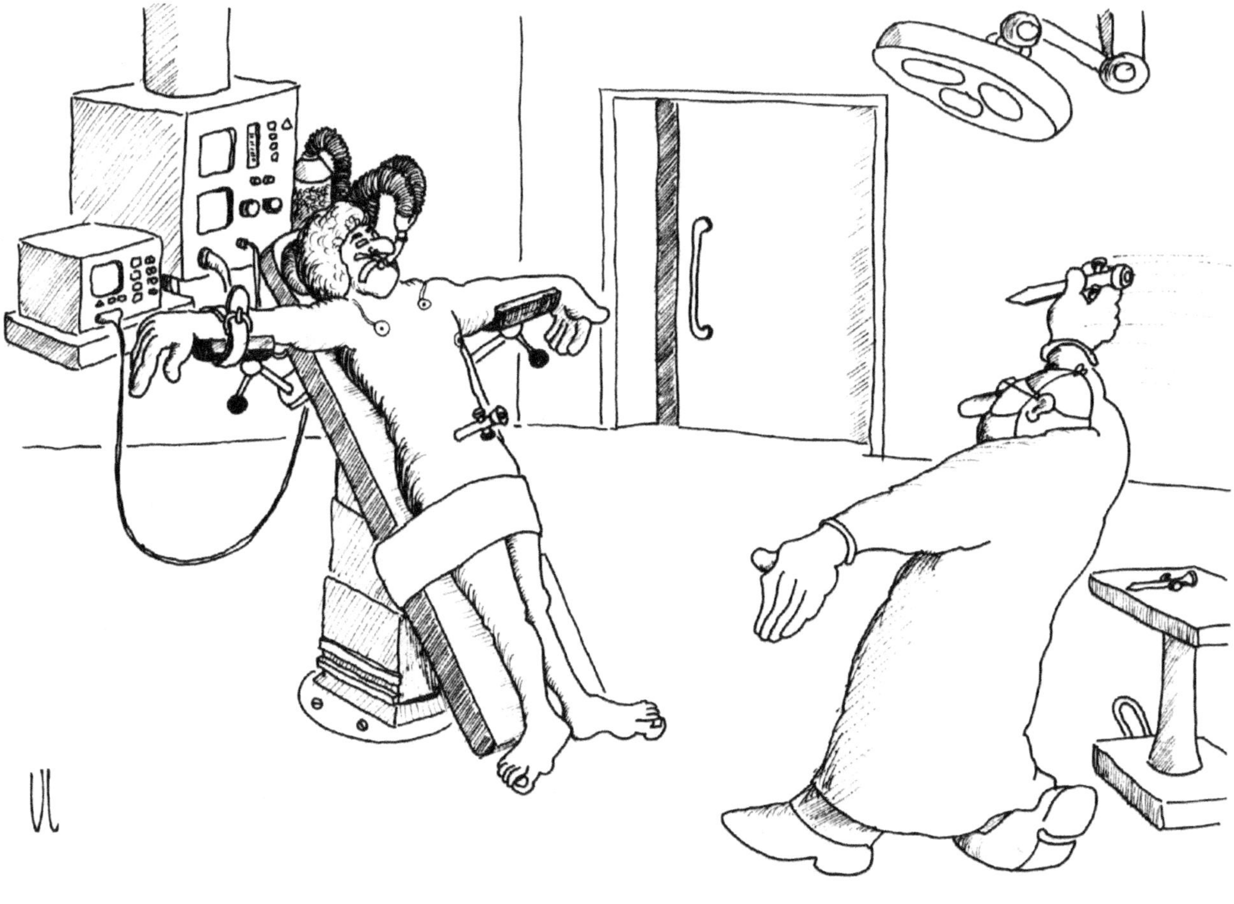

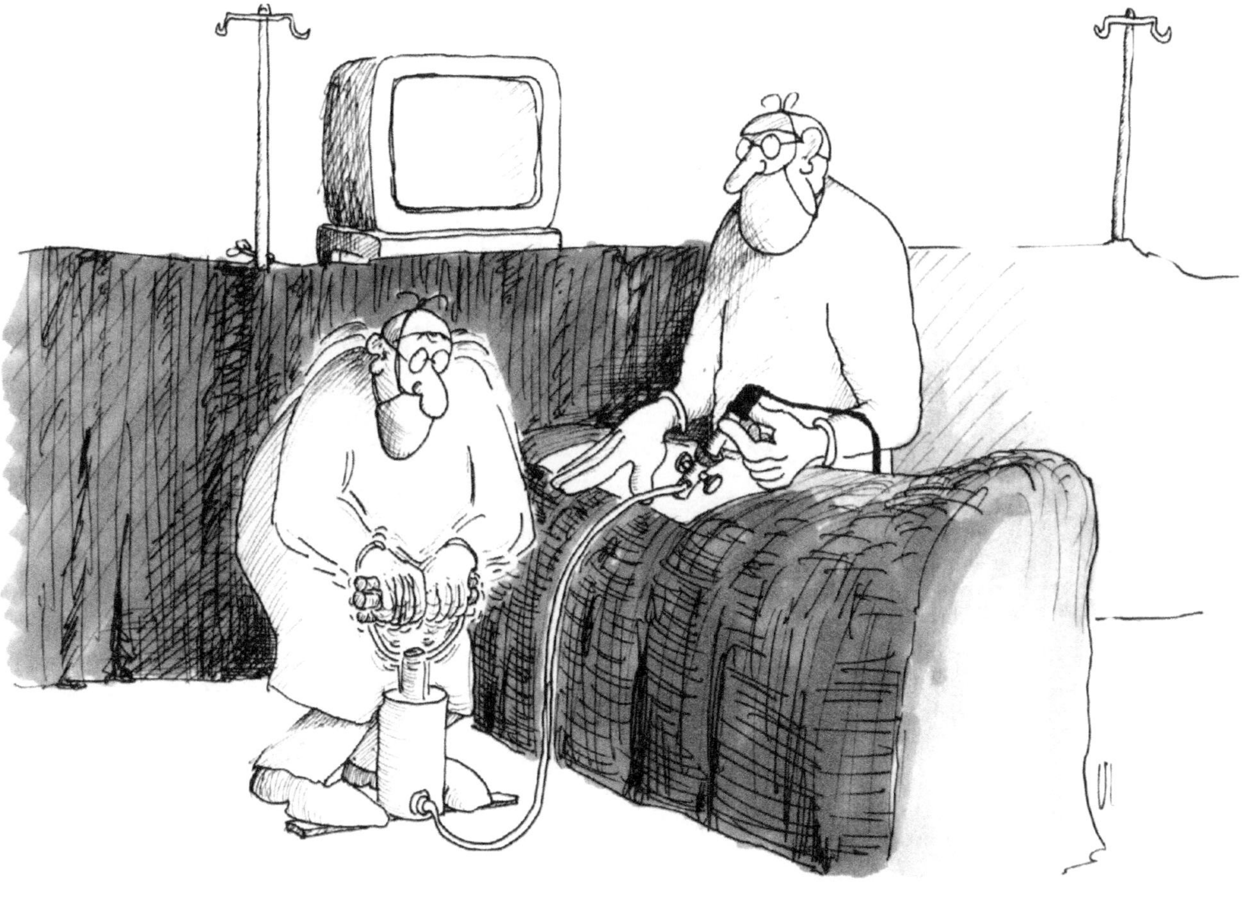

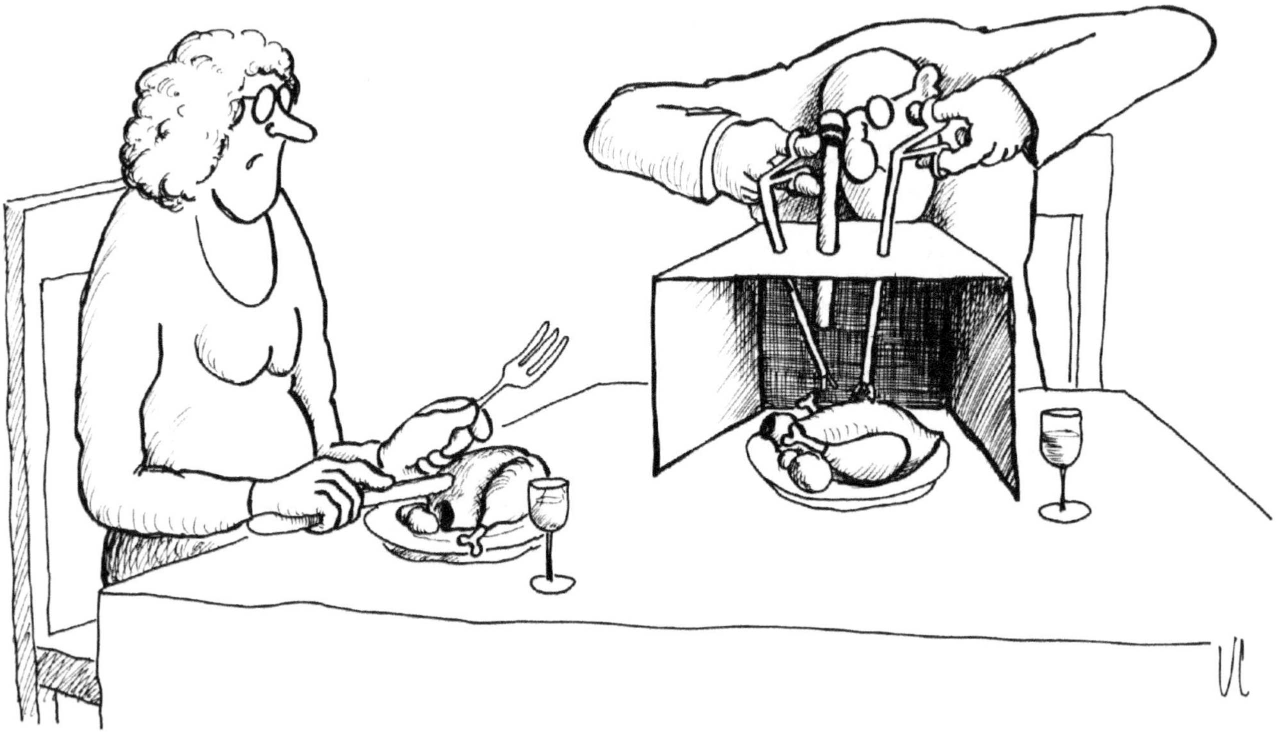

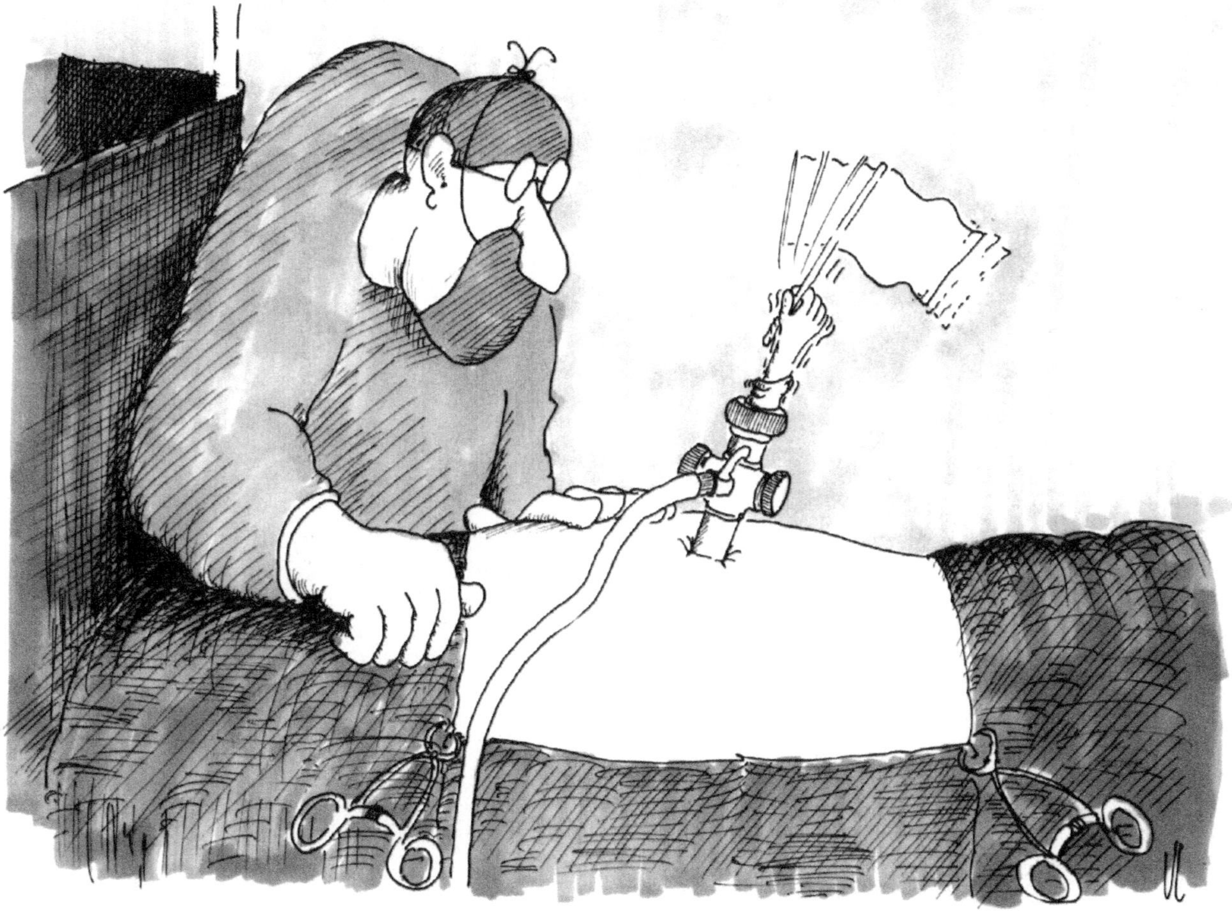

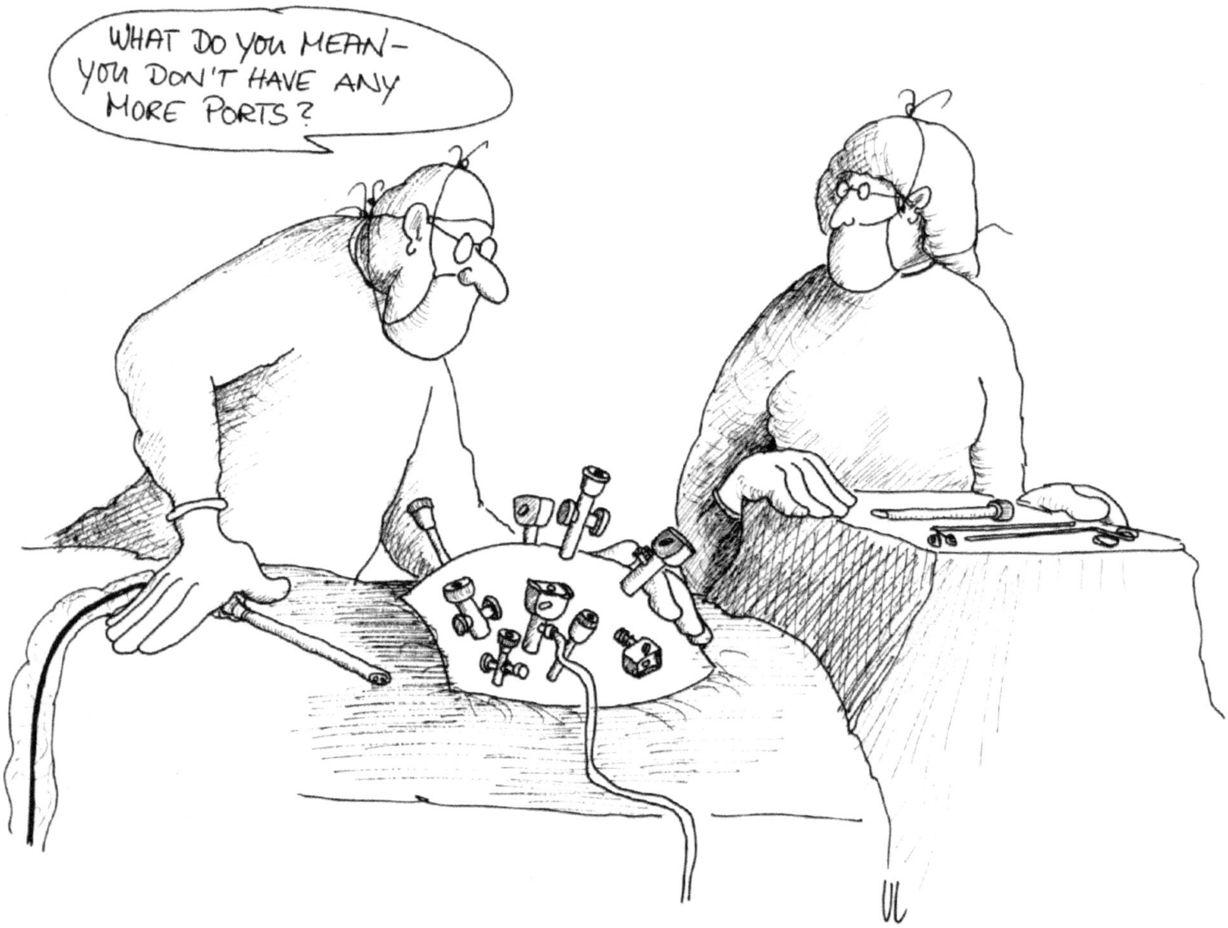
WHAT DO YOU MEAN - YOU DON'T HAVE ANY MORE PORTS?
UL

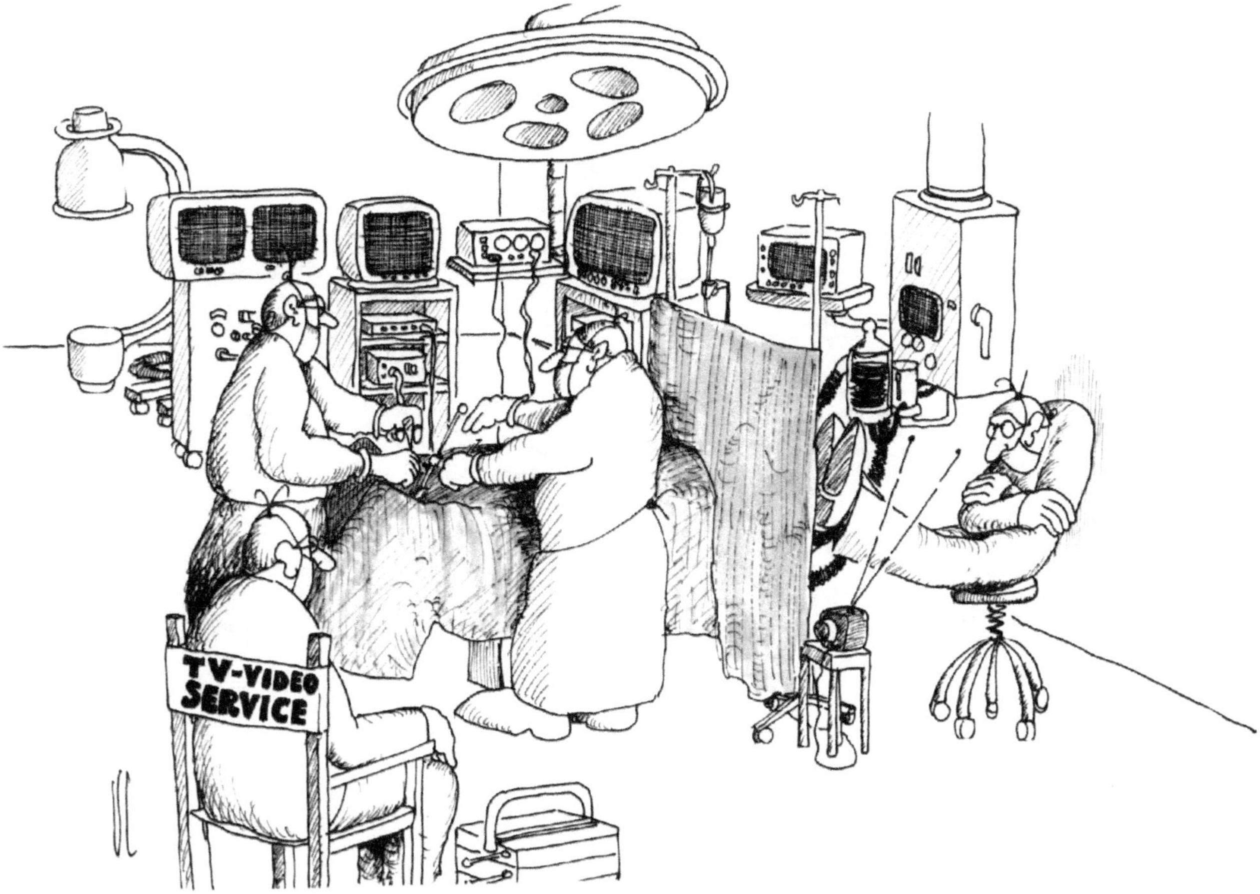
TV-VIDEO
SERVICE

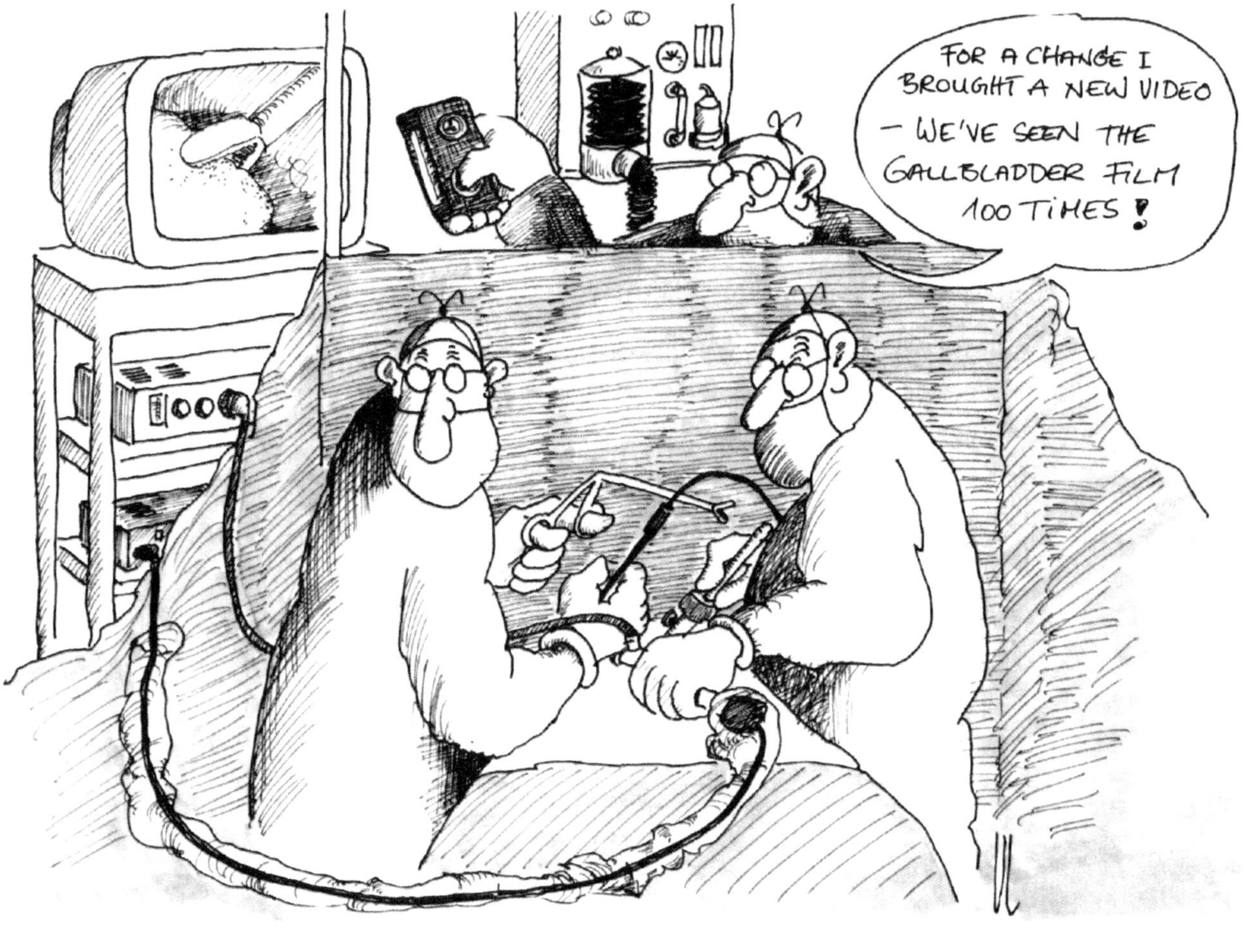
FOR A CHANGE I BROUGHT A NEW VIDEO – WE'VE SEEN THE GALLBLADDER FILM 100 TIMES!

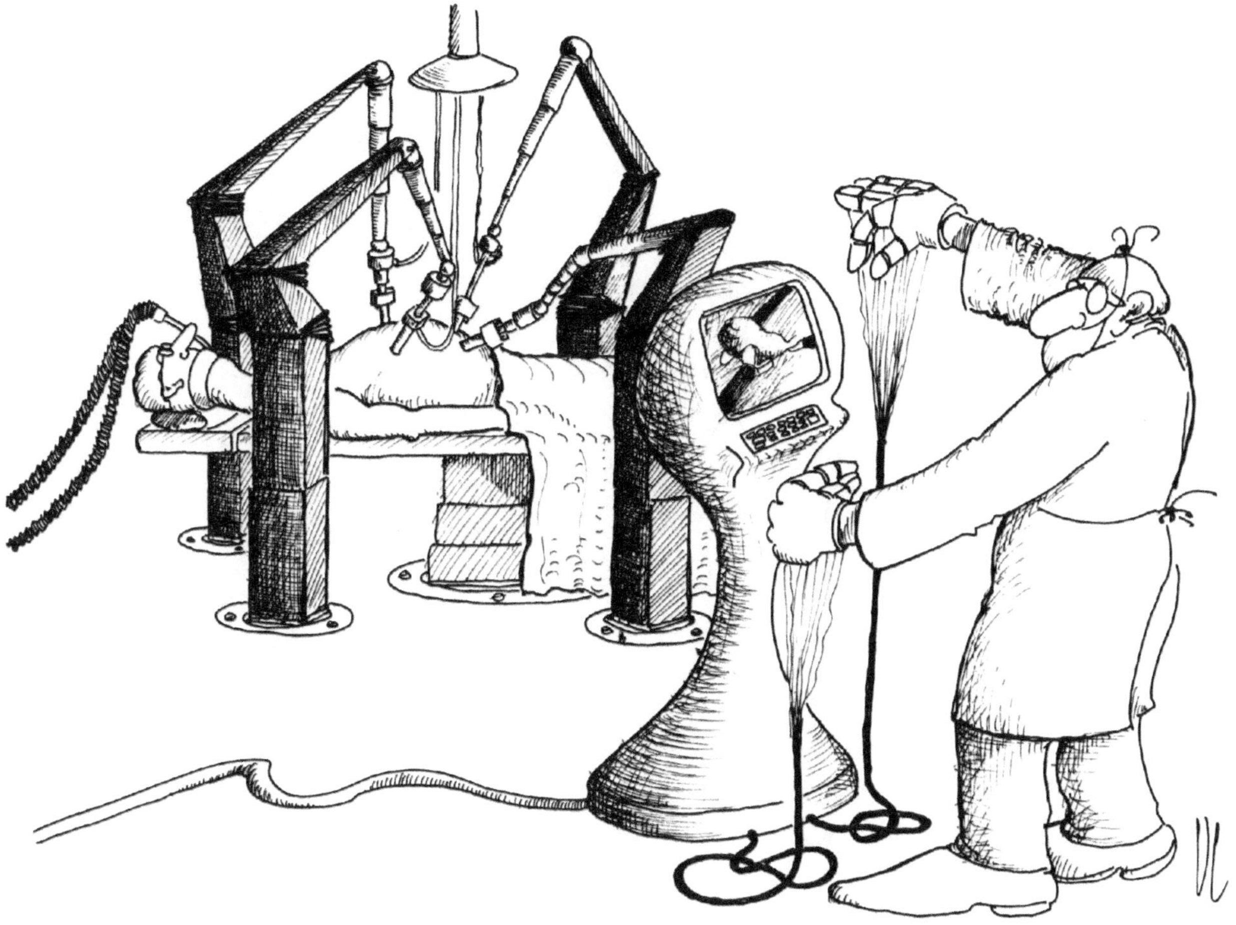

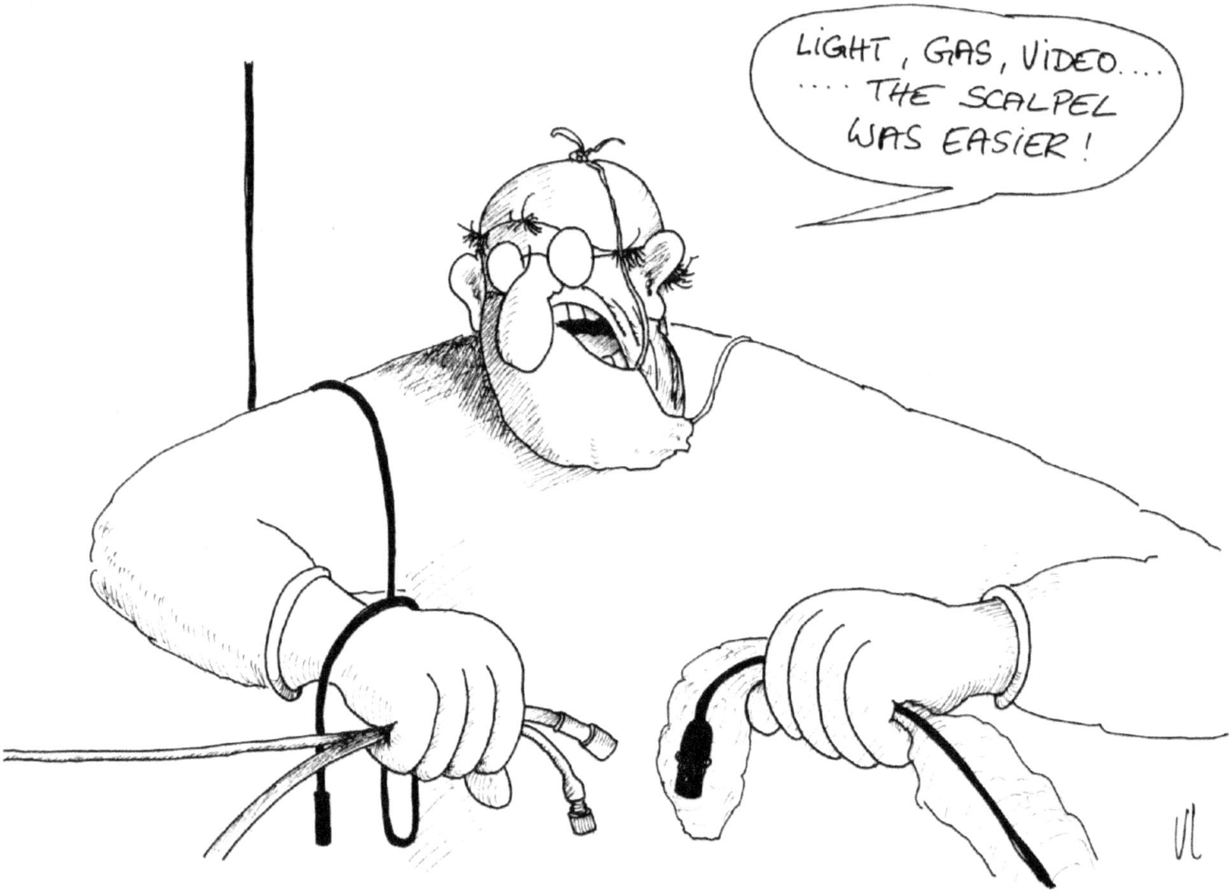
LIGHT, GAS, VIDEO.... ....THE SCALPEL WAS EASIER!

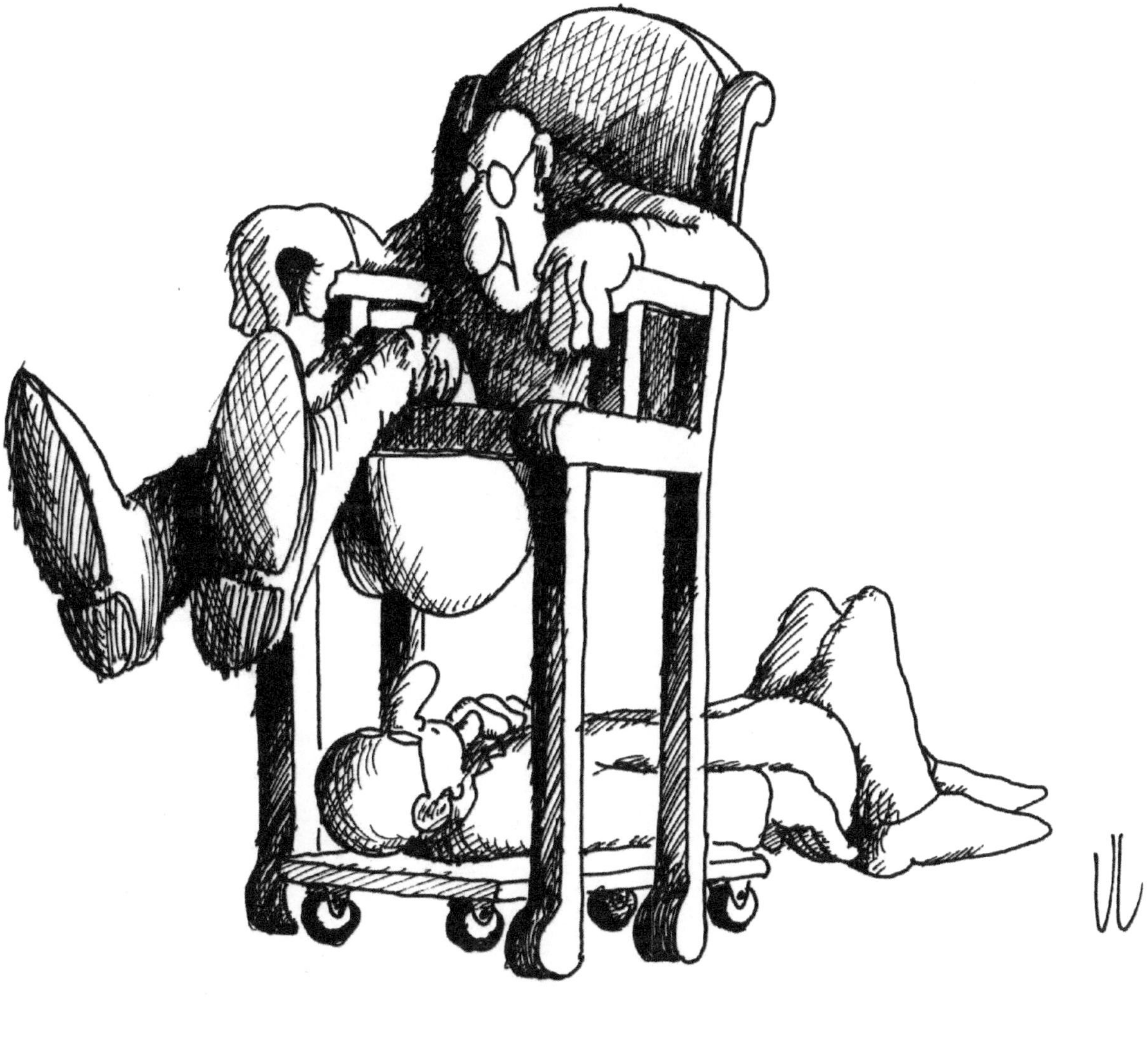

# DERMA-TOLOGY

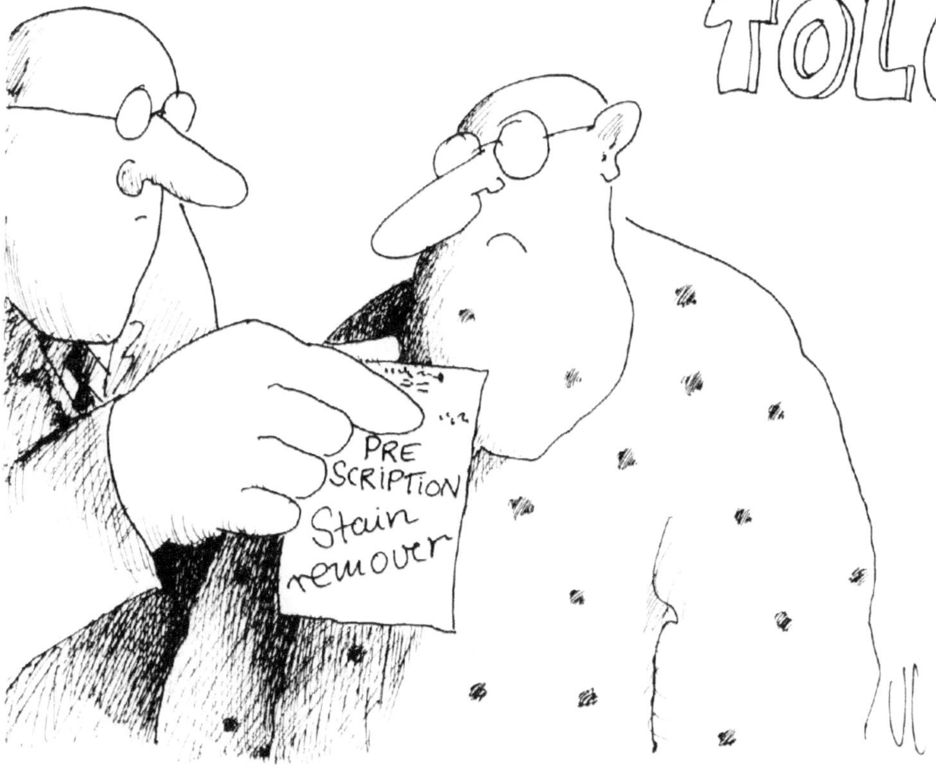

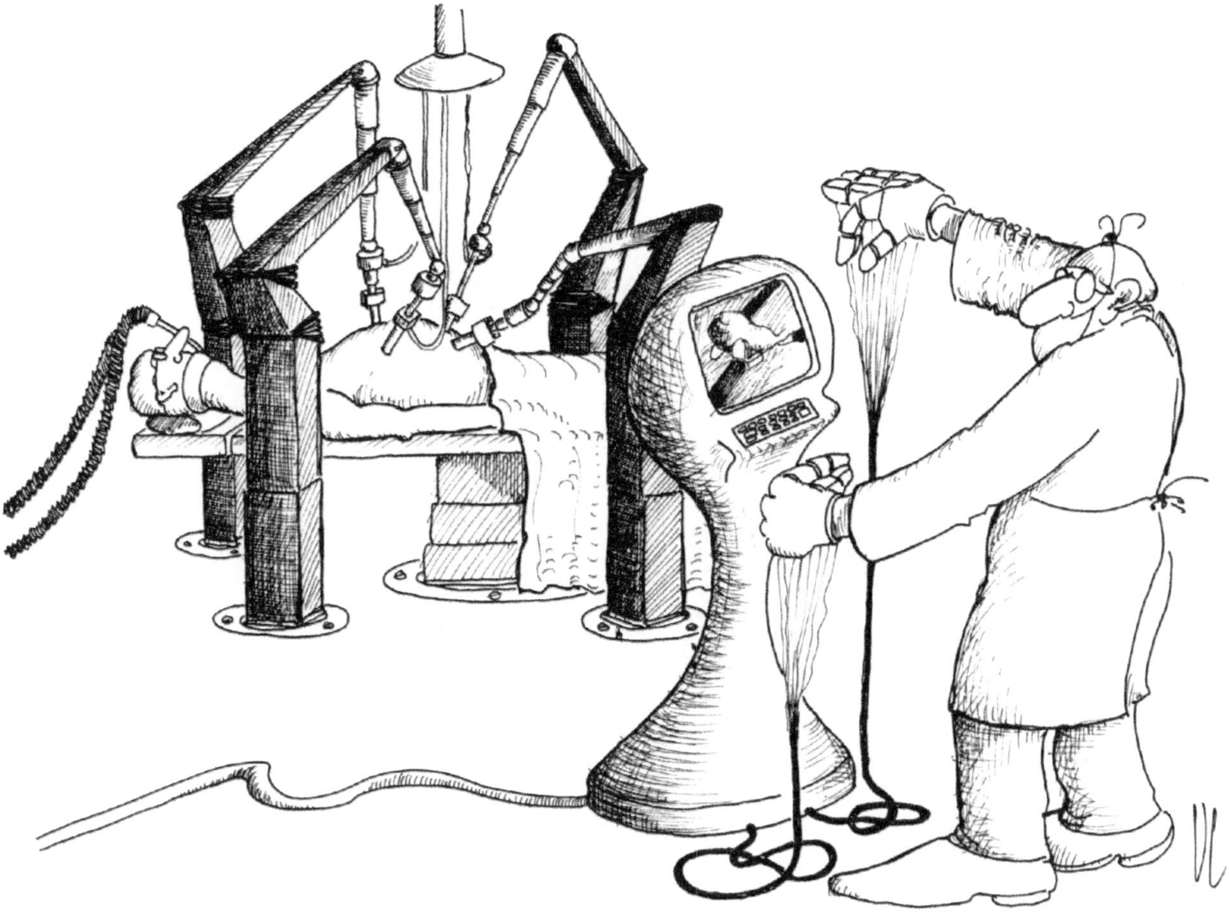

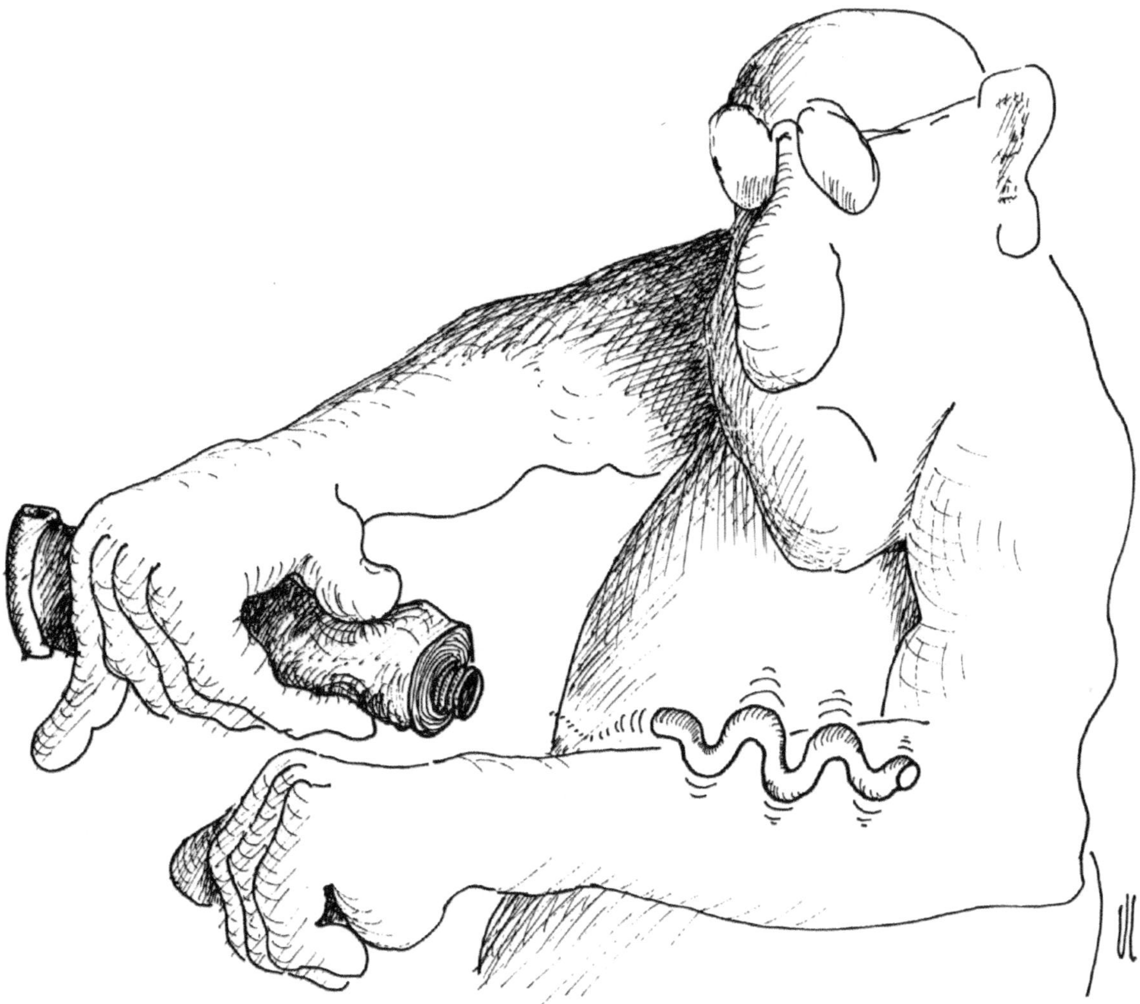

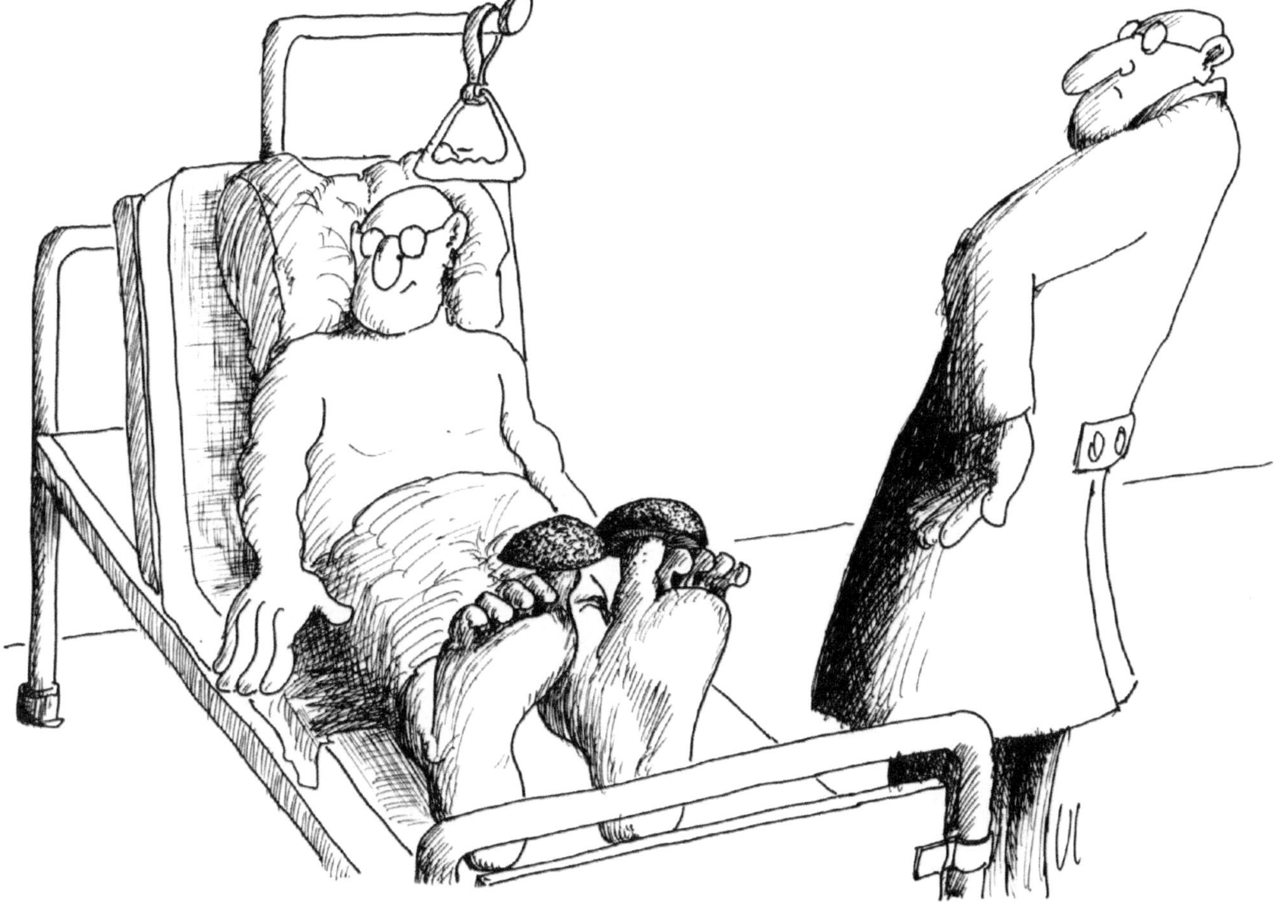

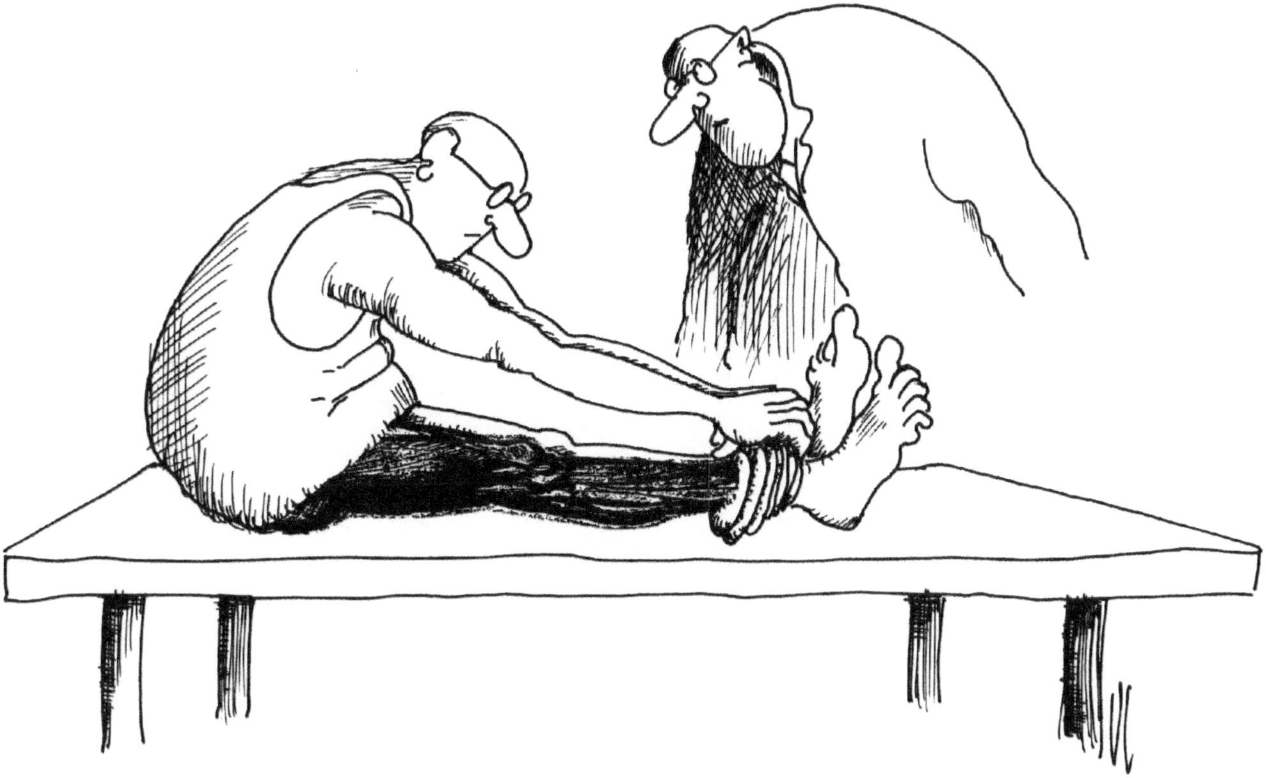

# ENDOSCOPY

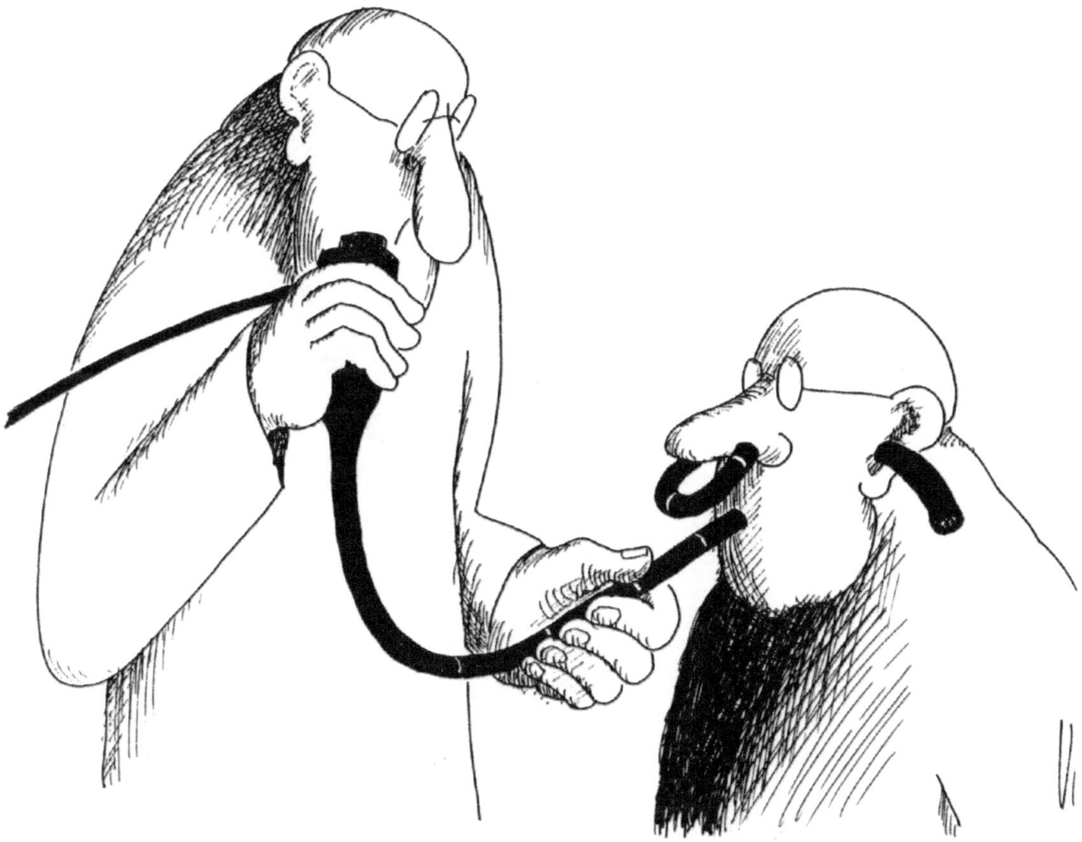

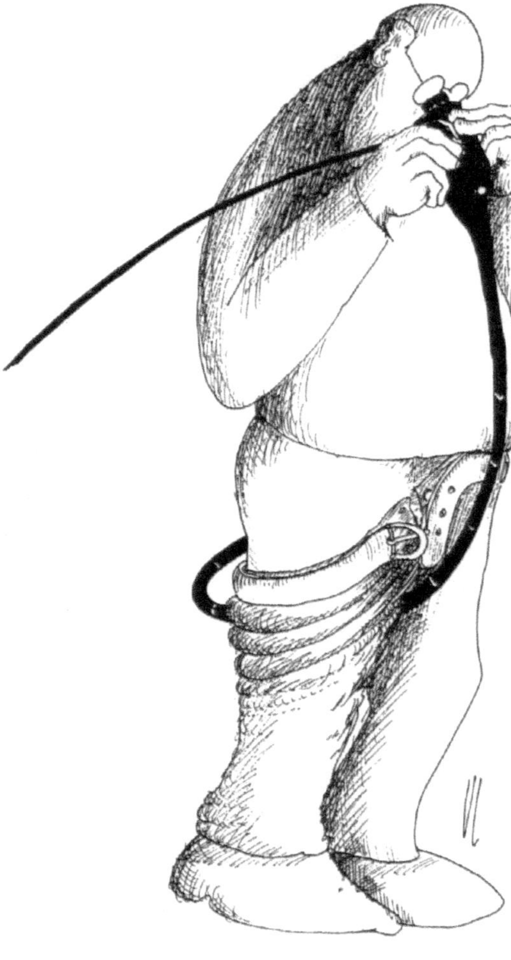

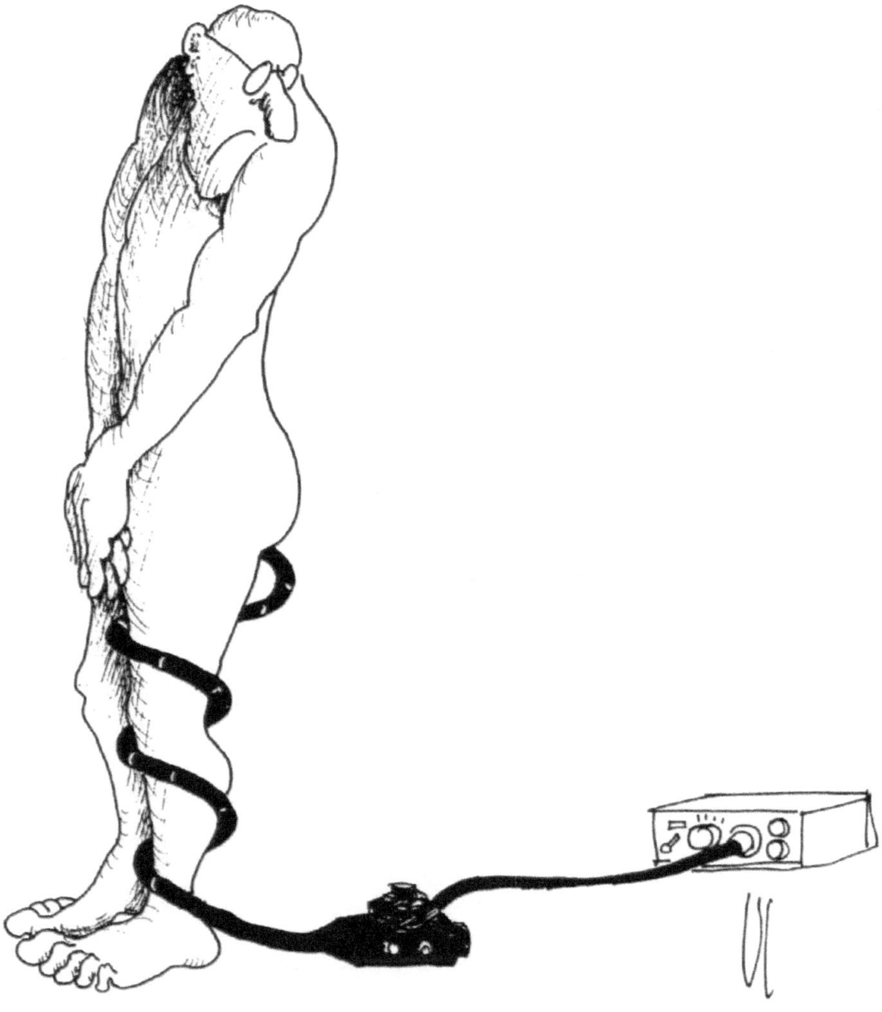

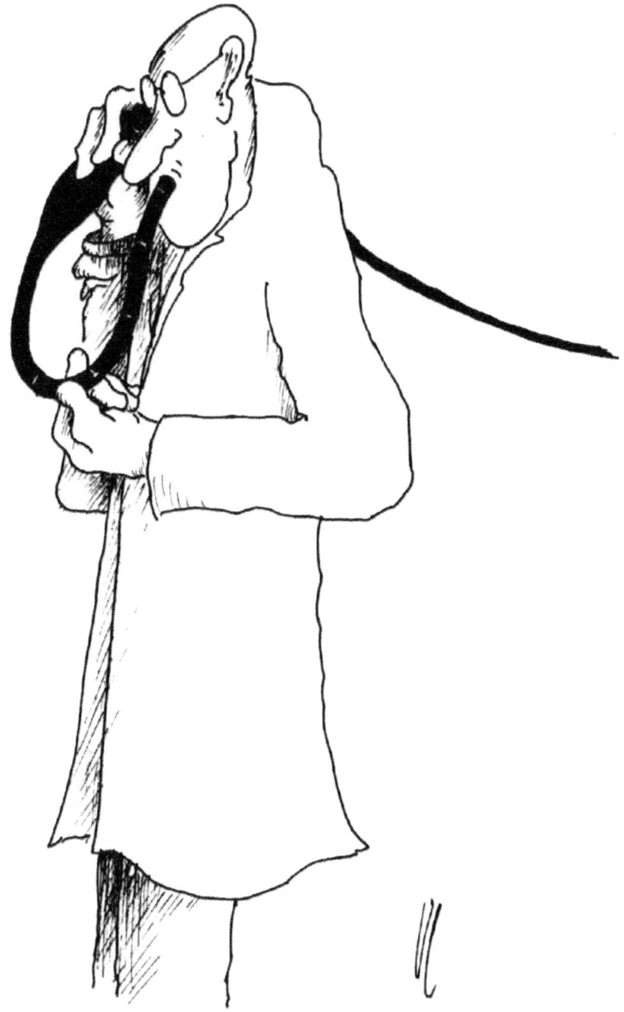

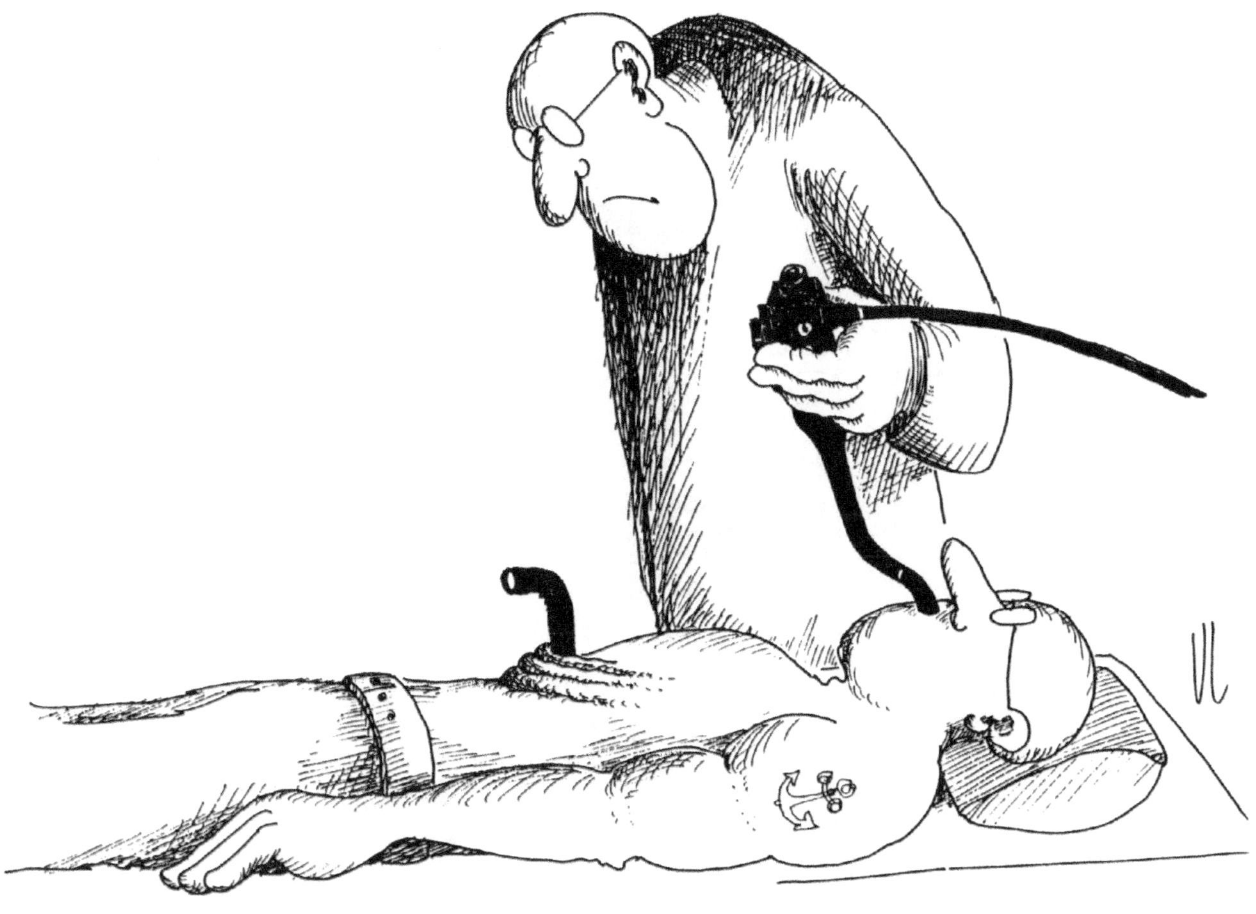

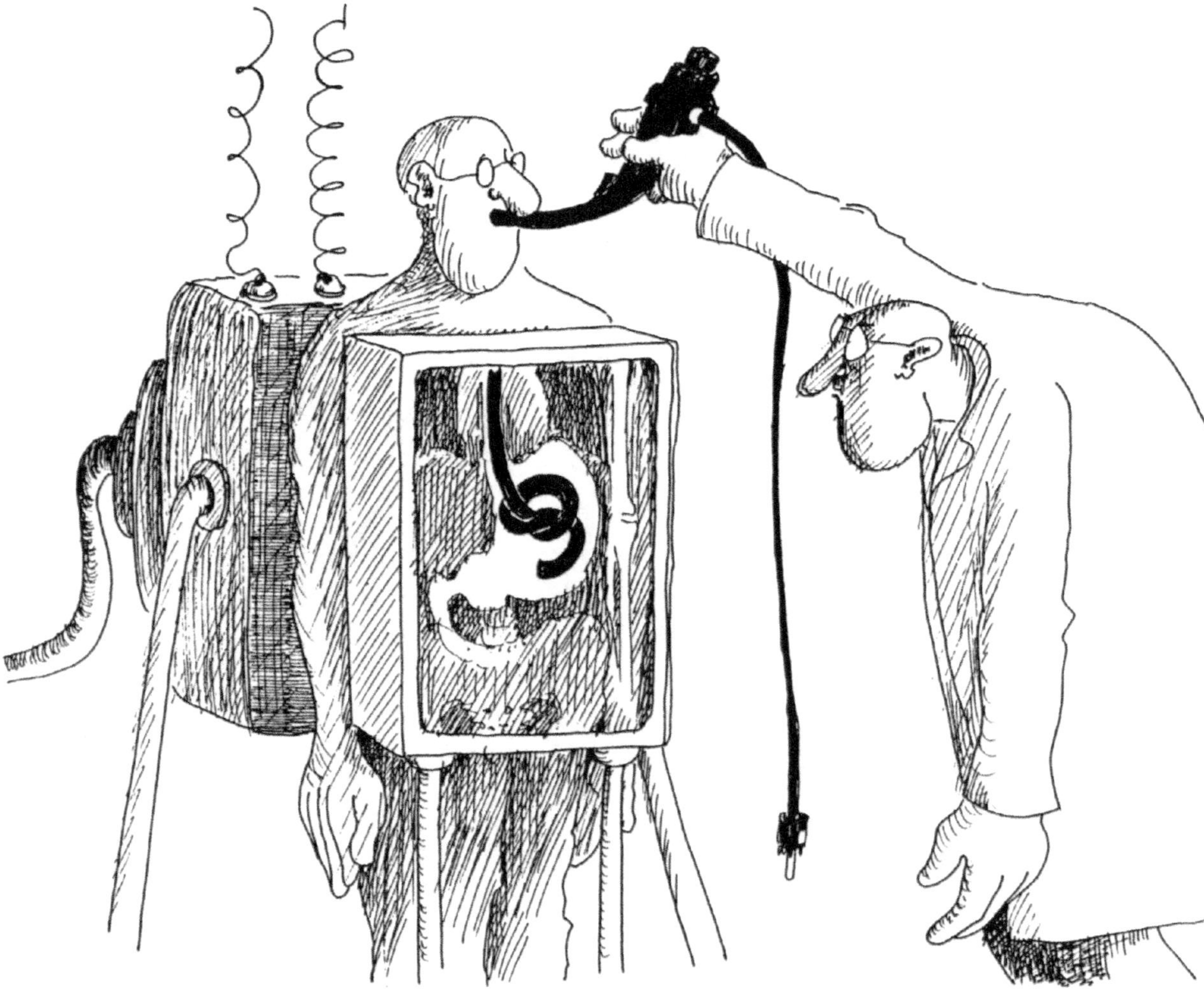

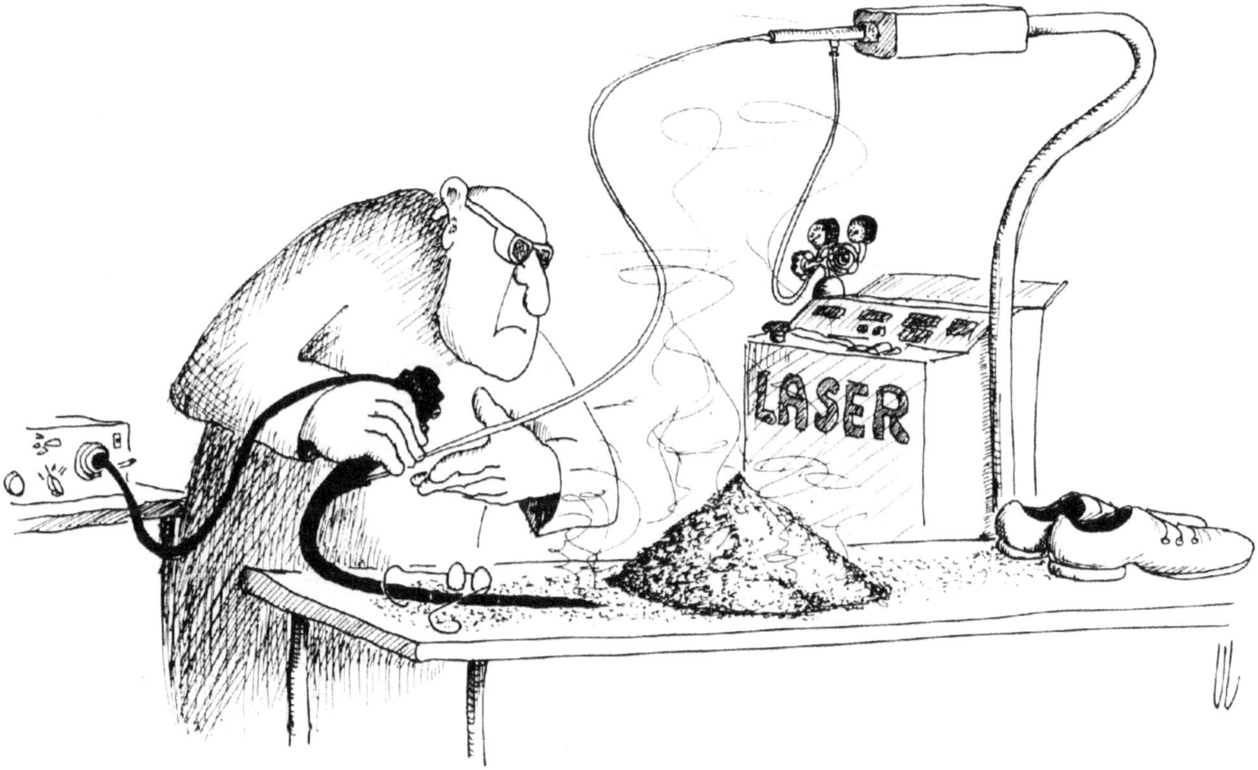
LASER

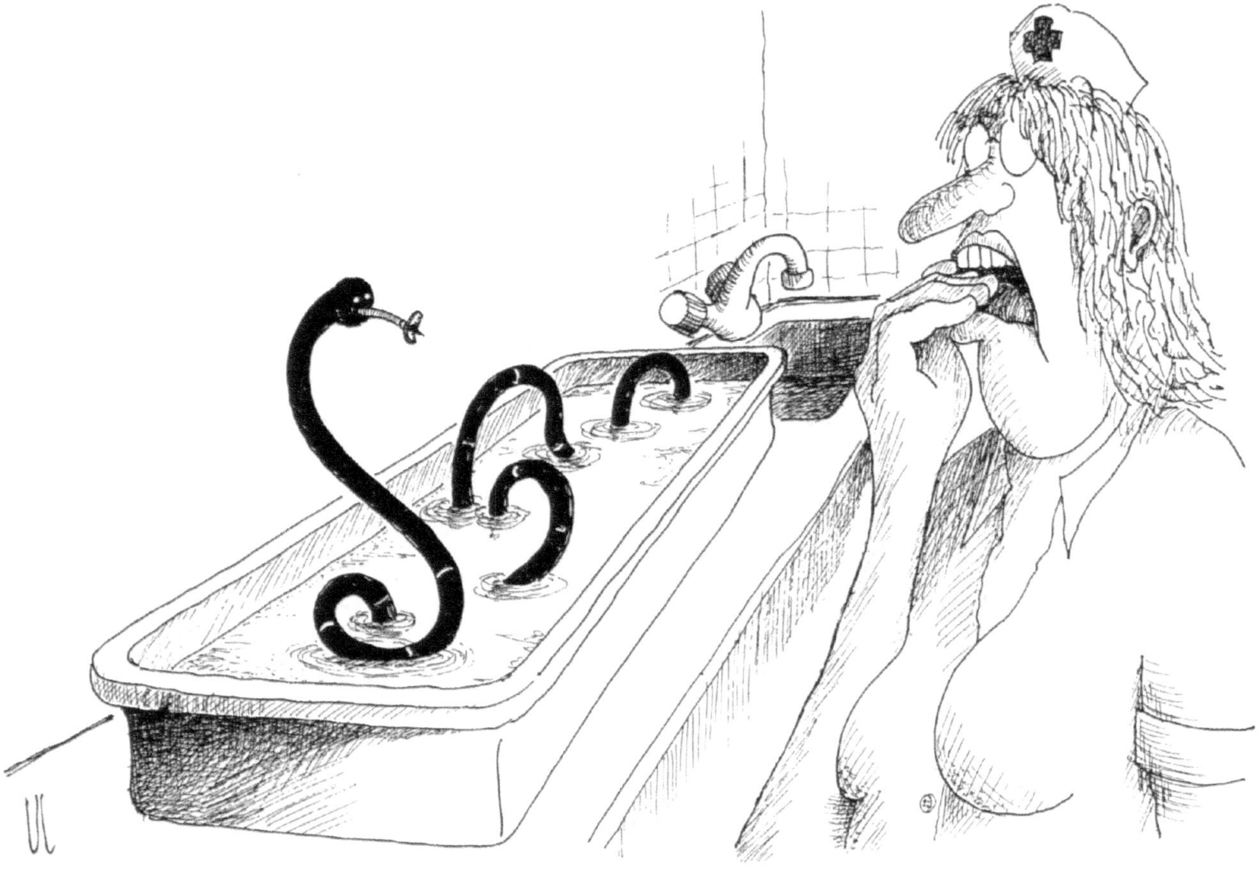

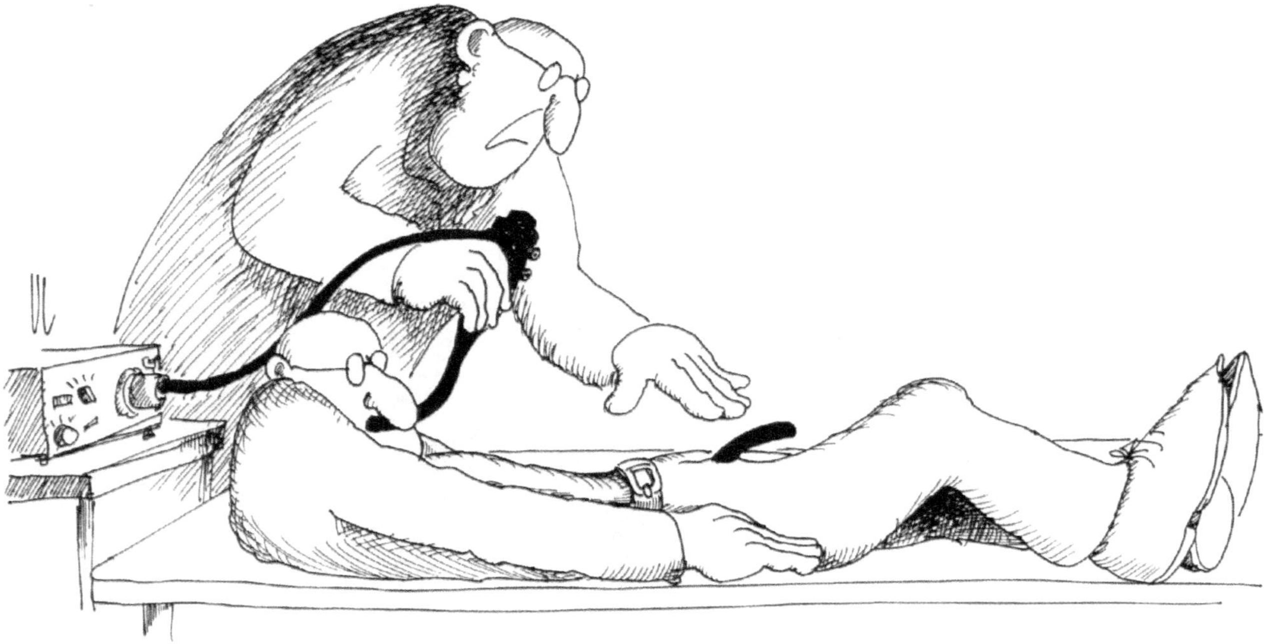

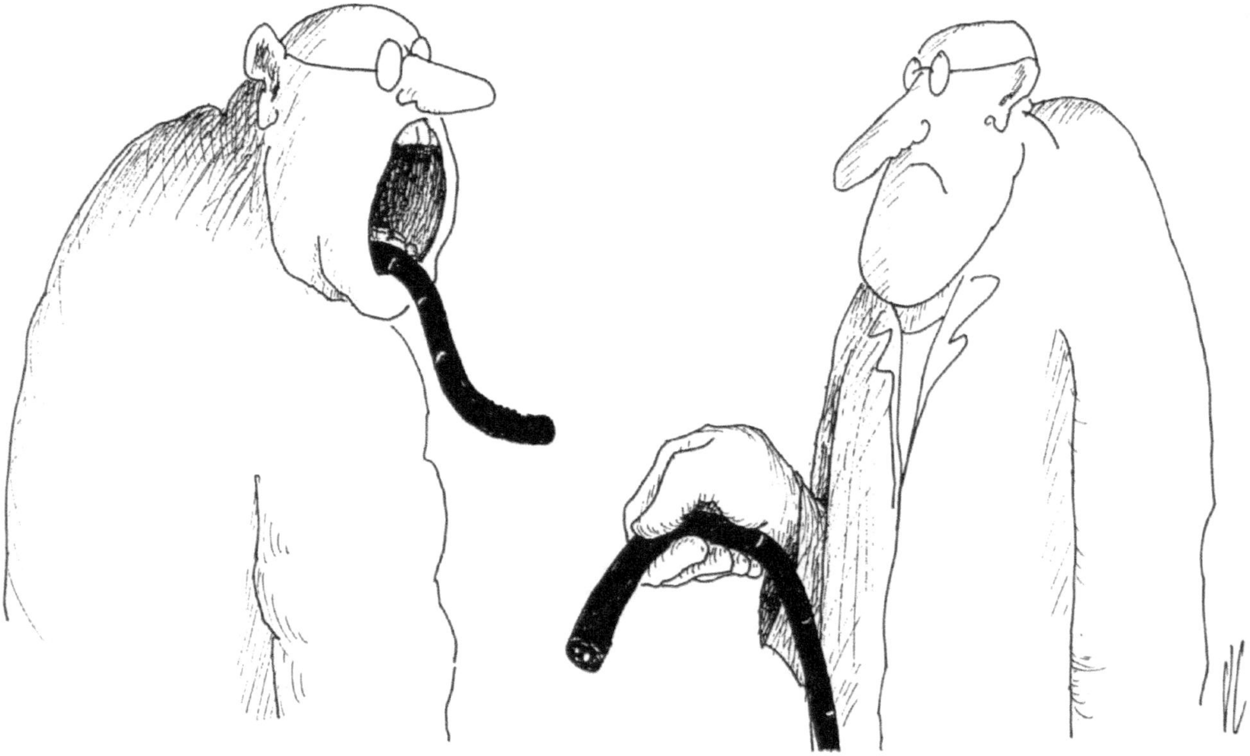

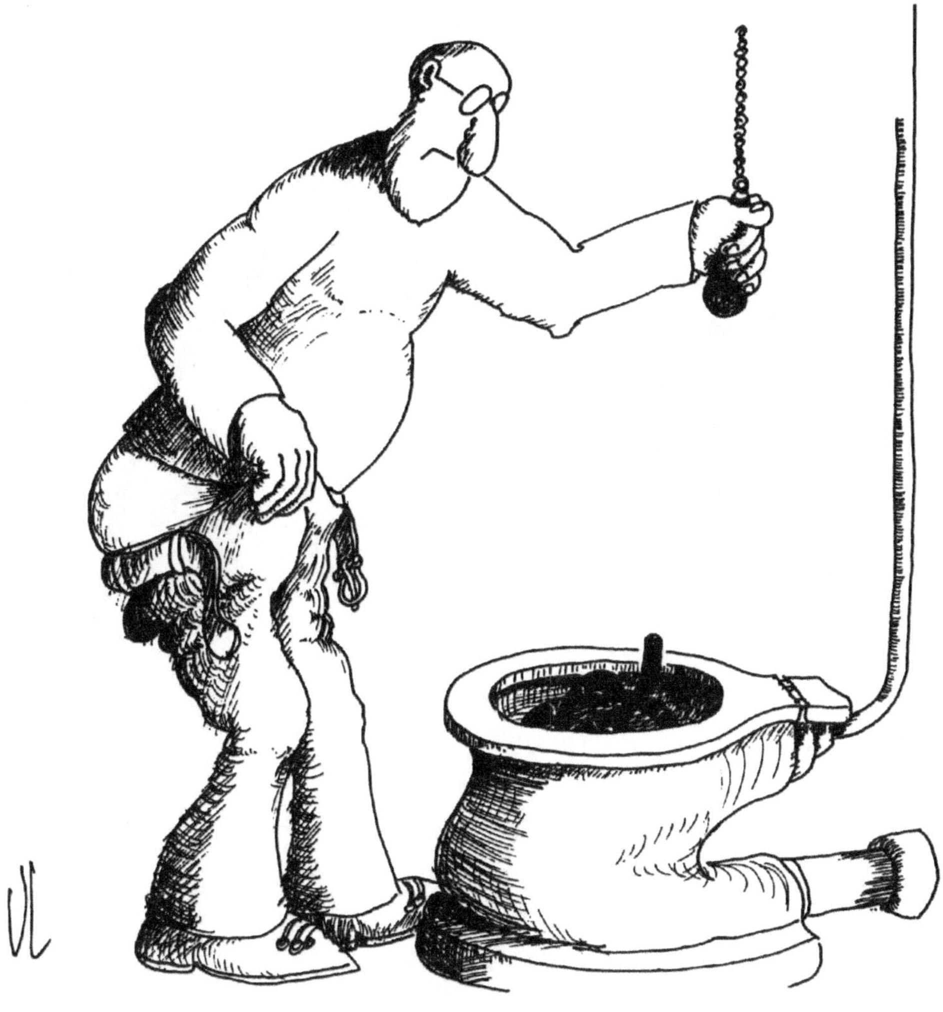

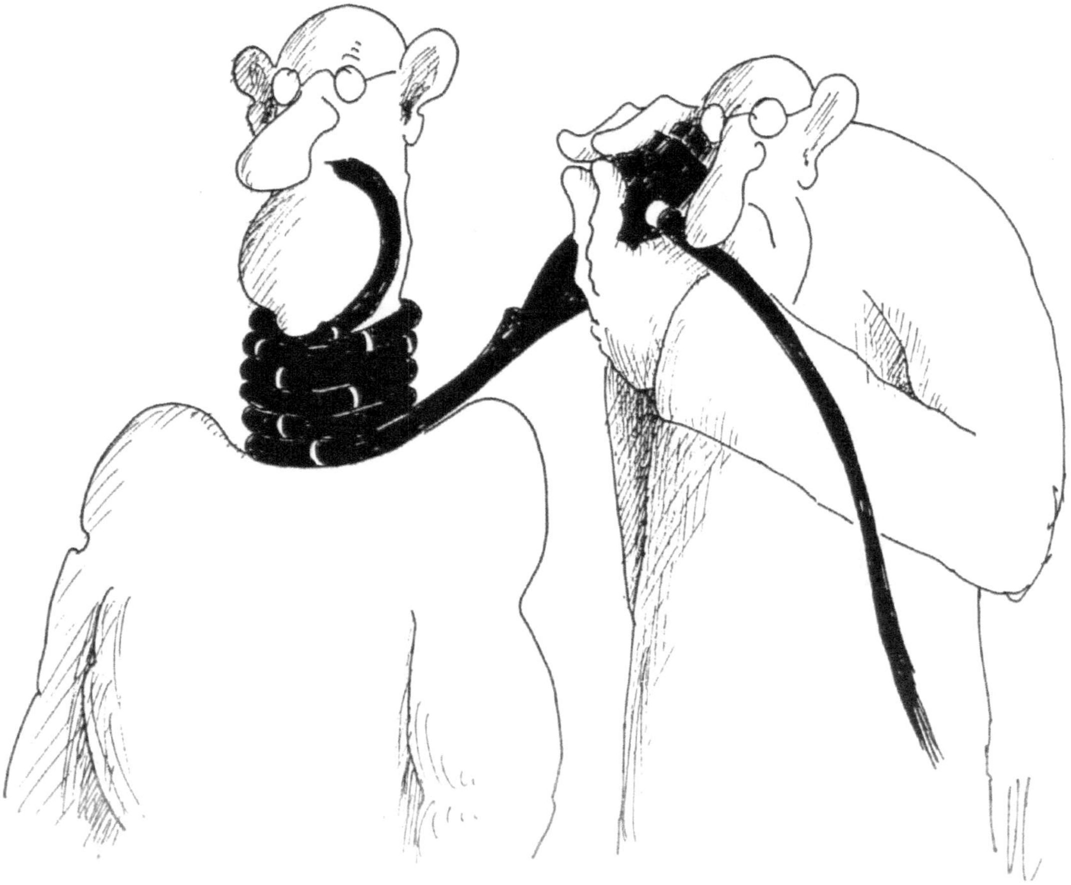

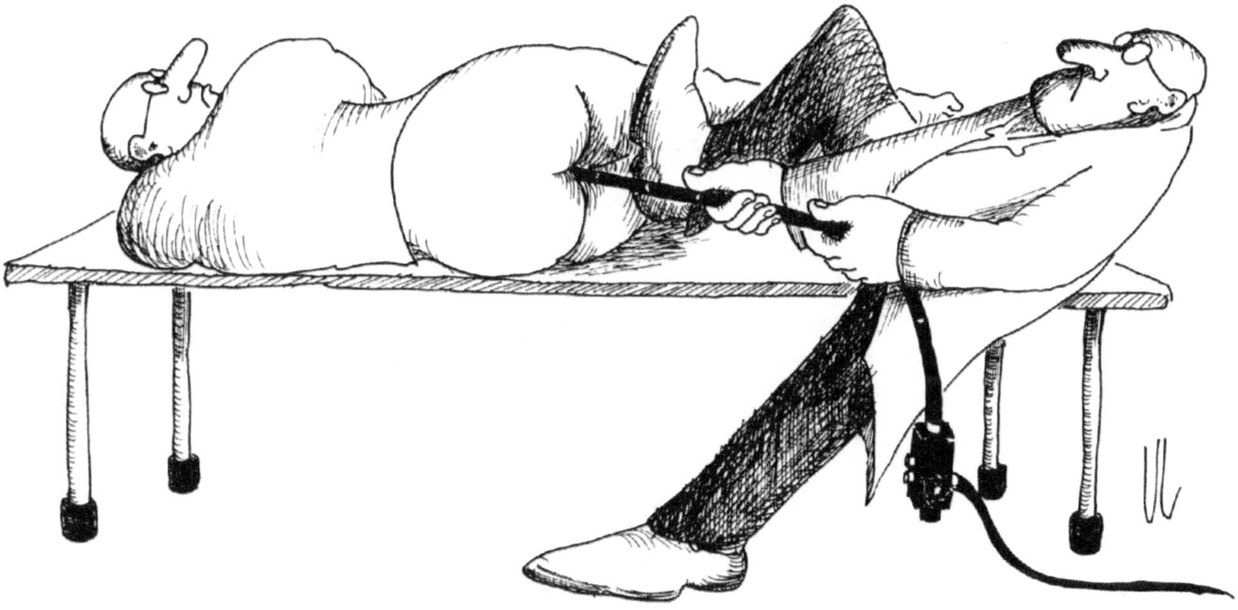

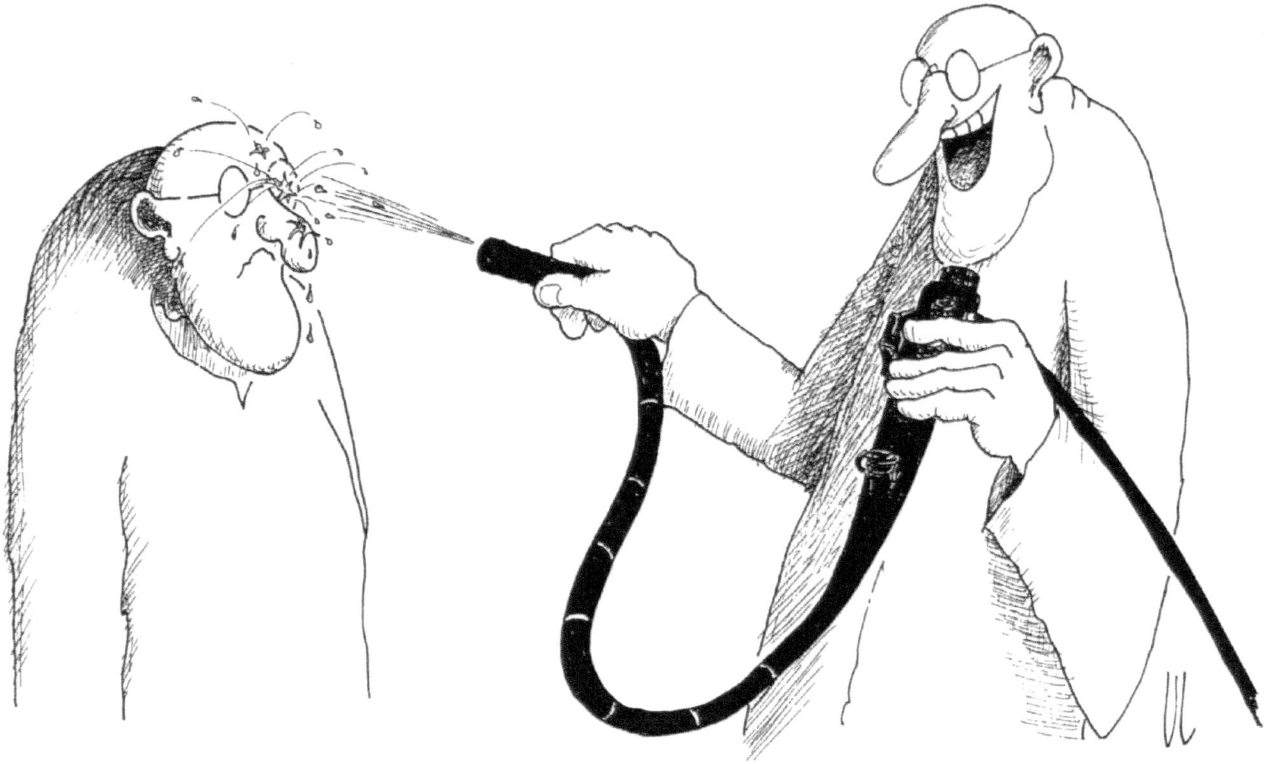

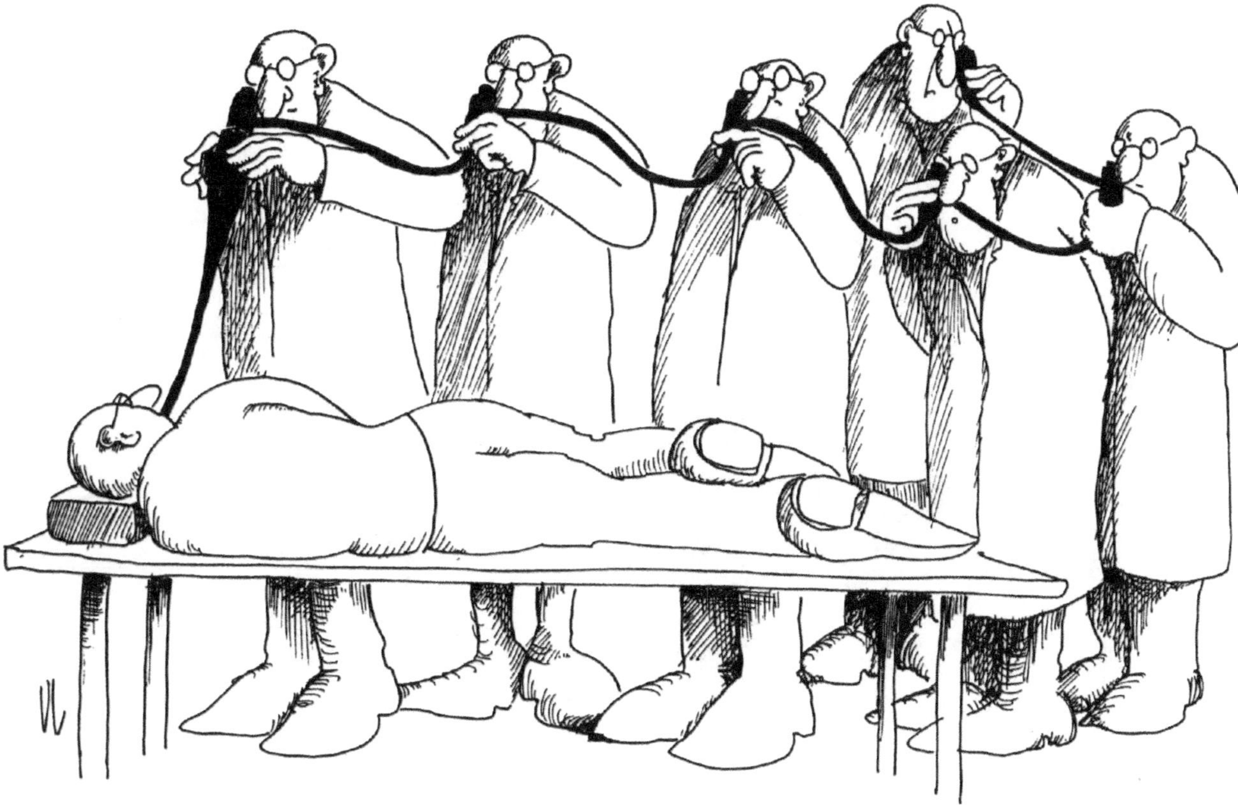

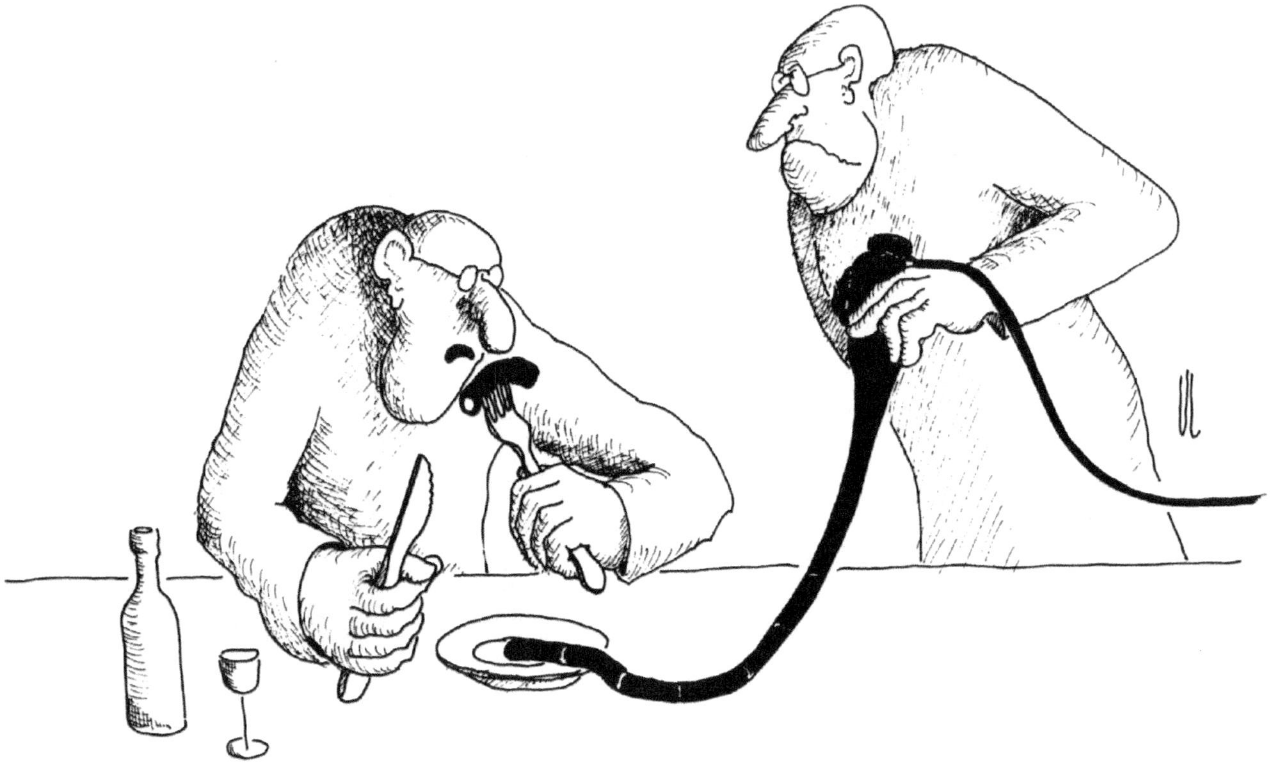

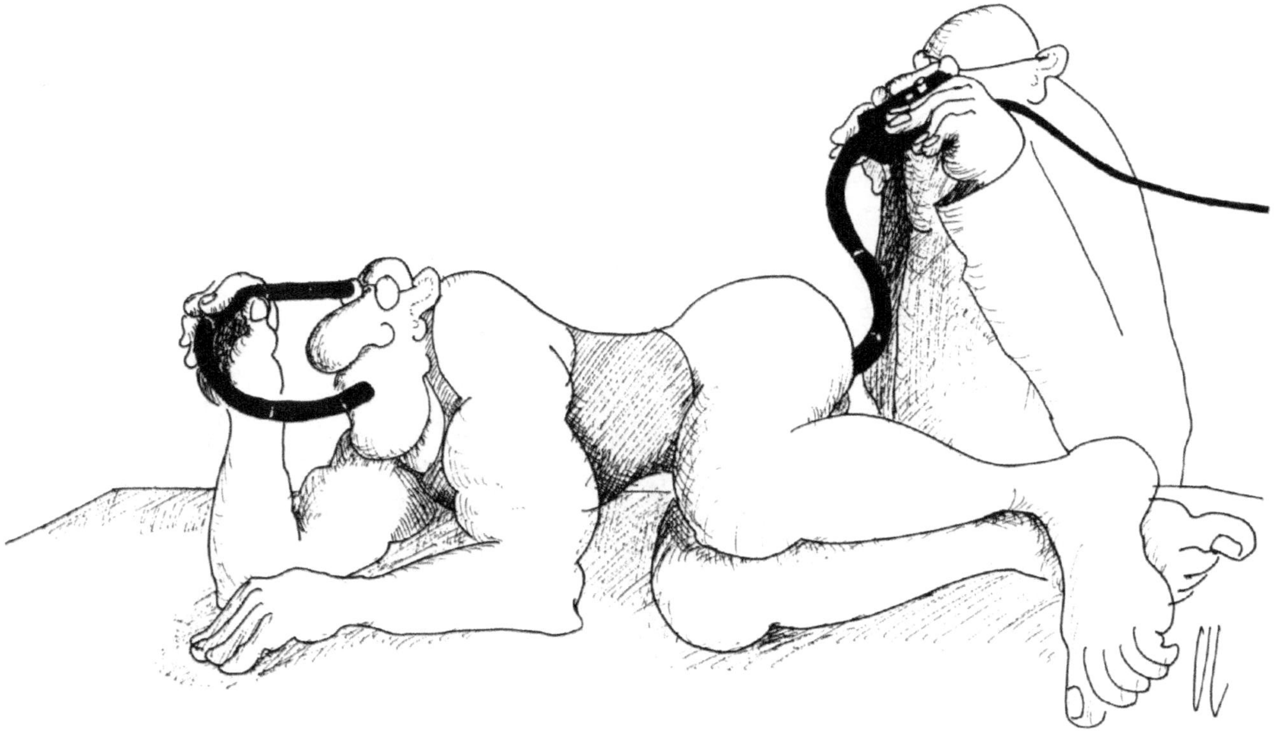

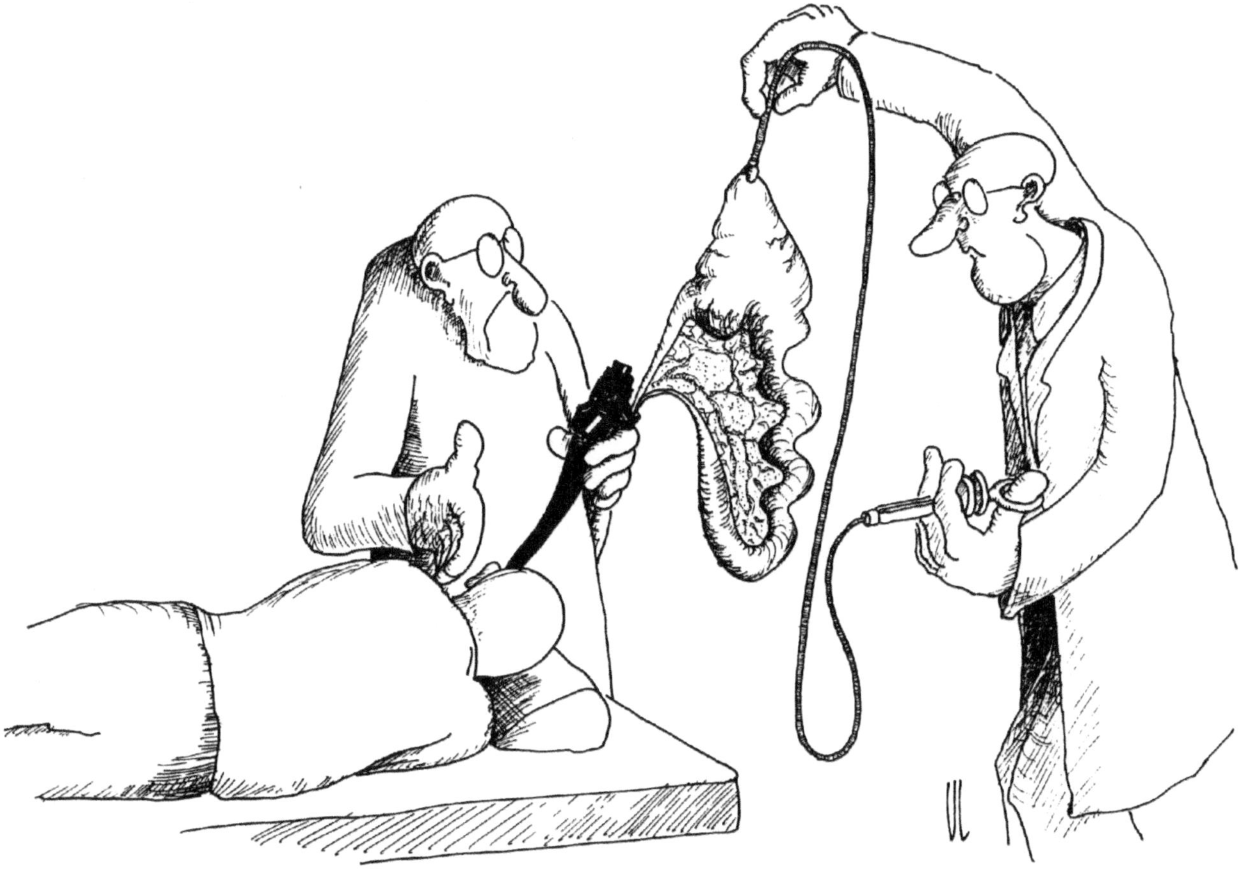

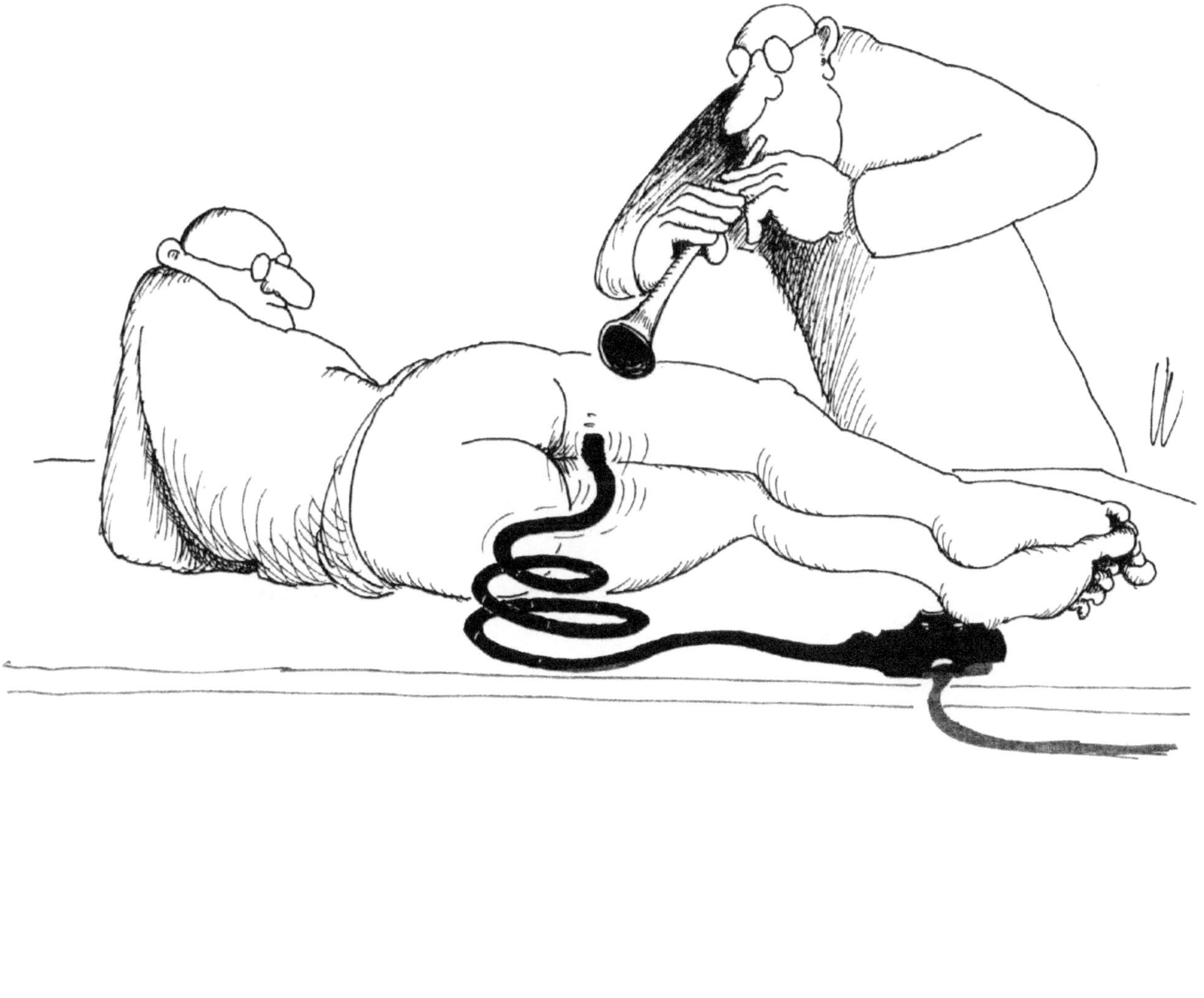

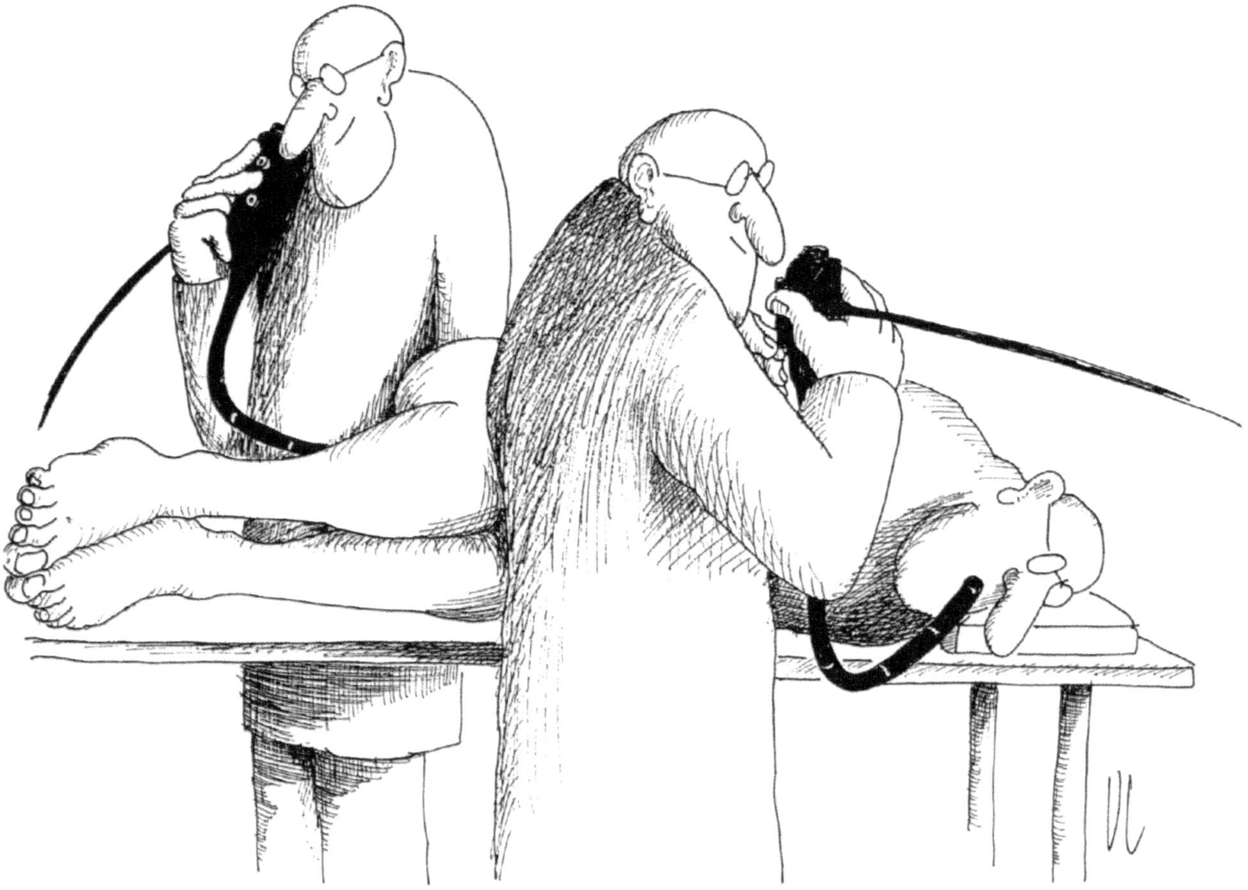

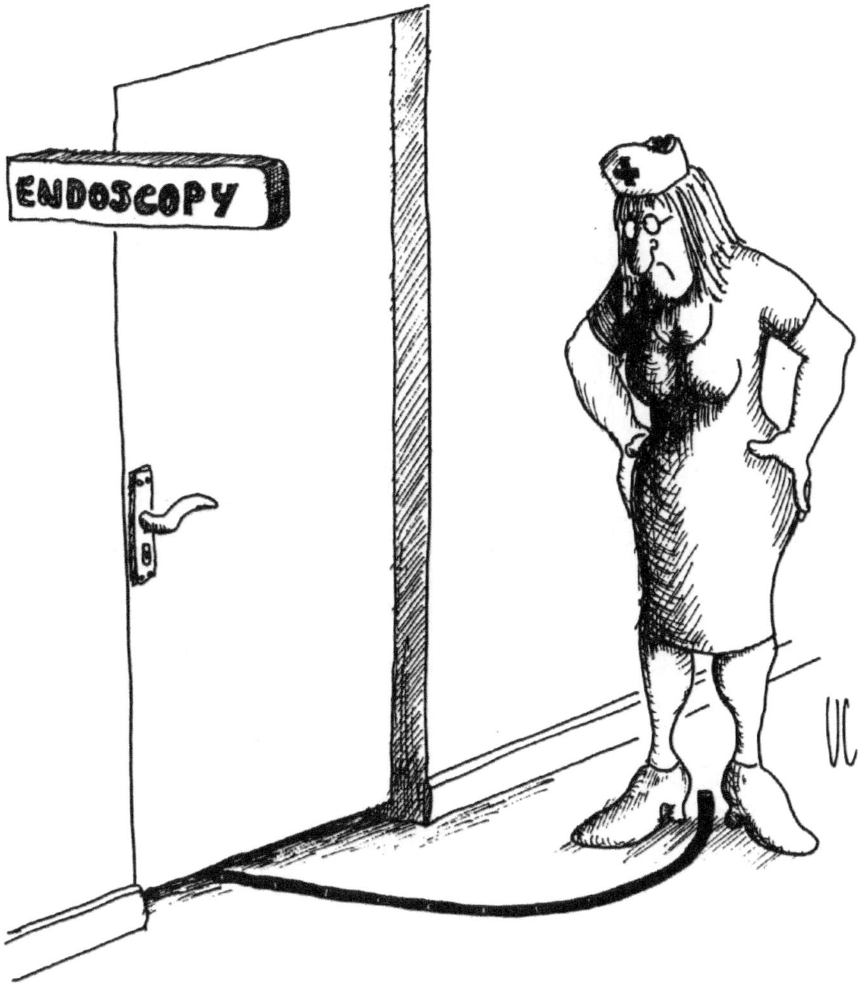
ENDOSCOPY
UC

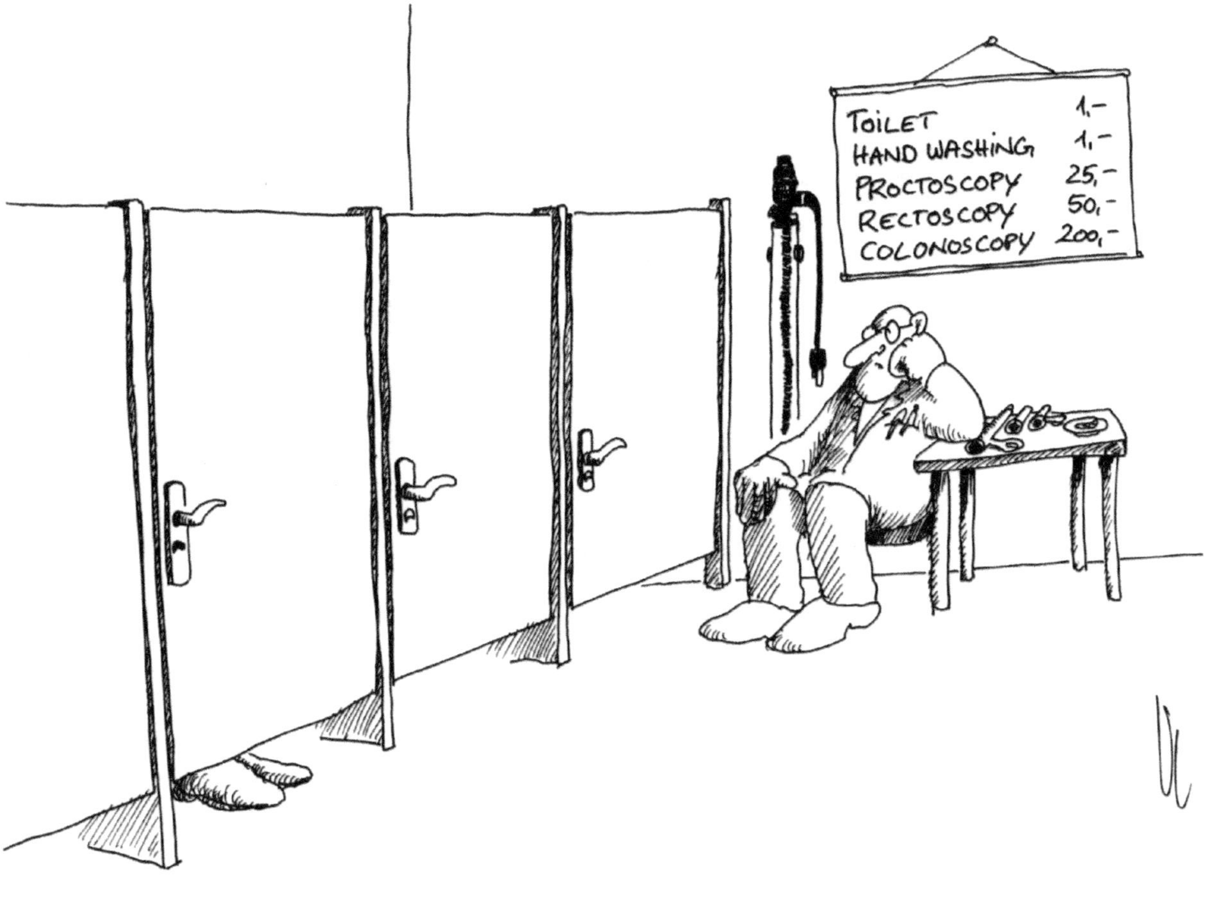
TOILET 1,-
HAND WASHING 1,-
PROCTOSCOPY 25,-
RECTOSCOPY 50,-
COLONOSCOPY 200,-

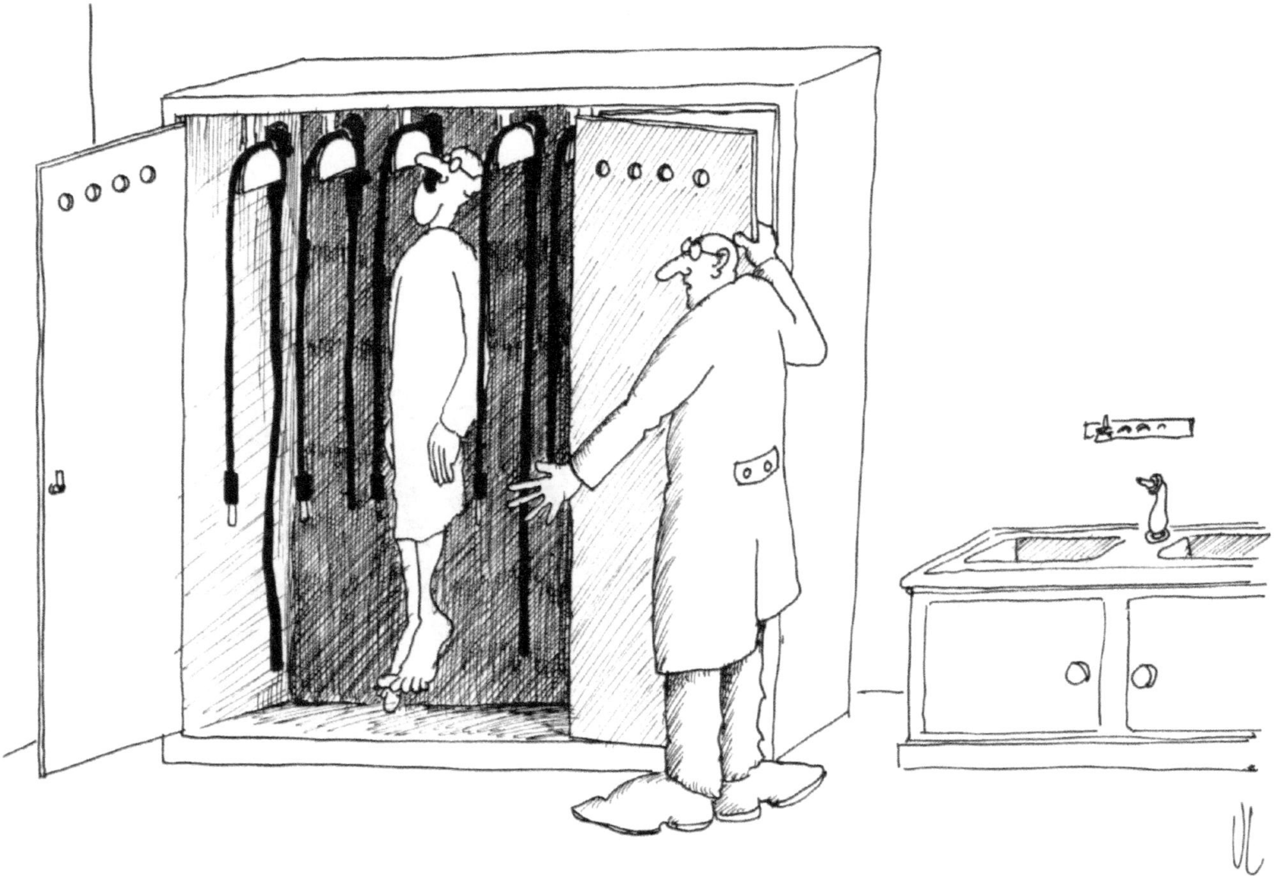

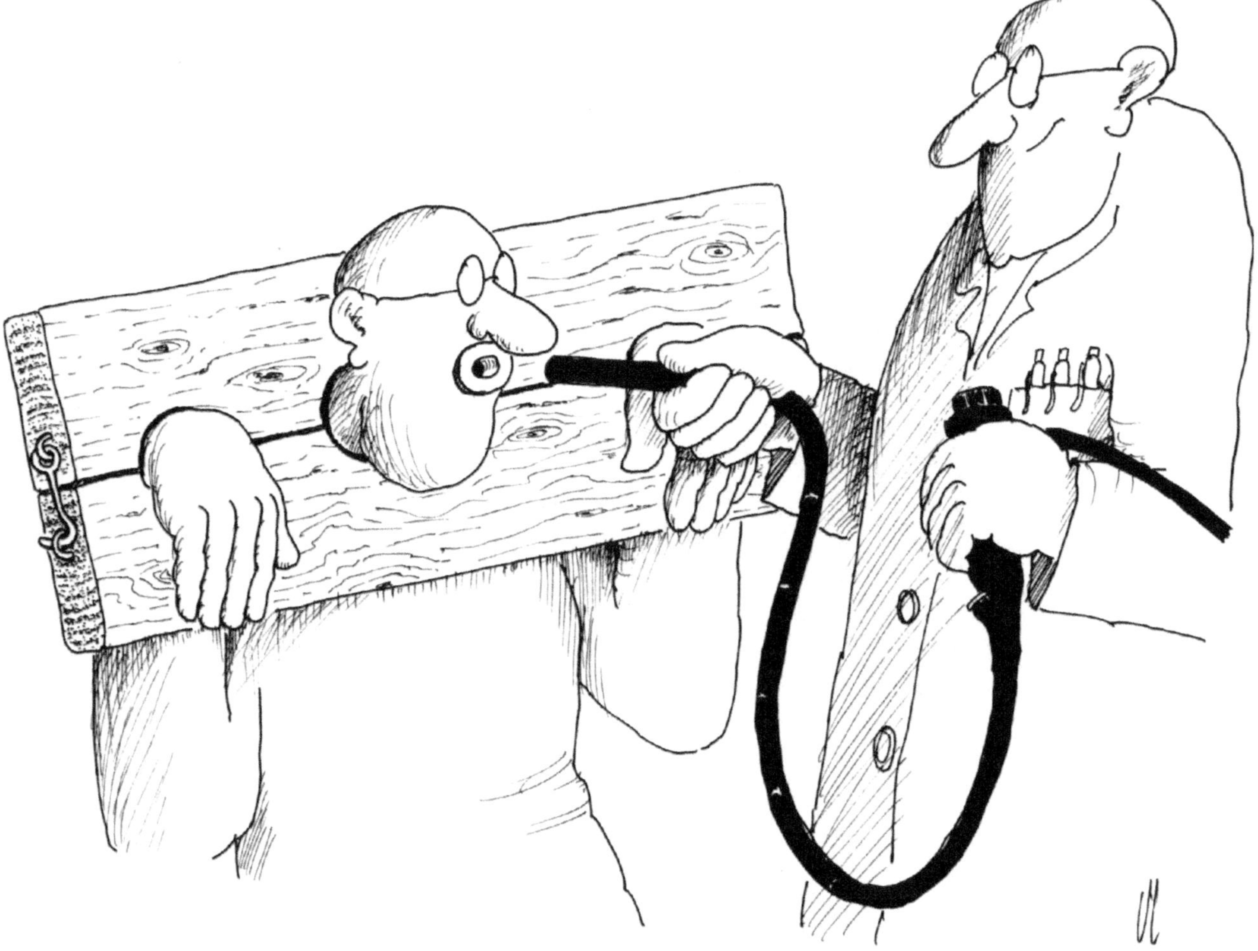

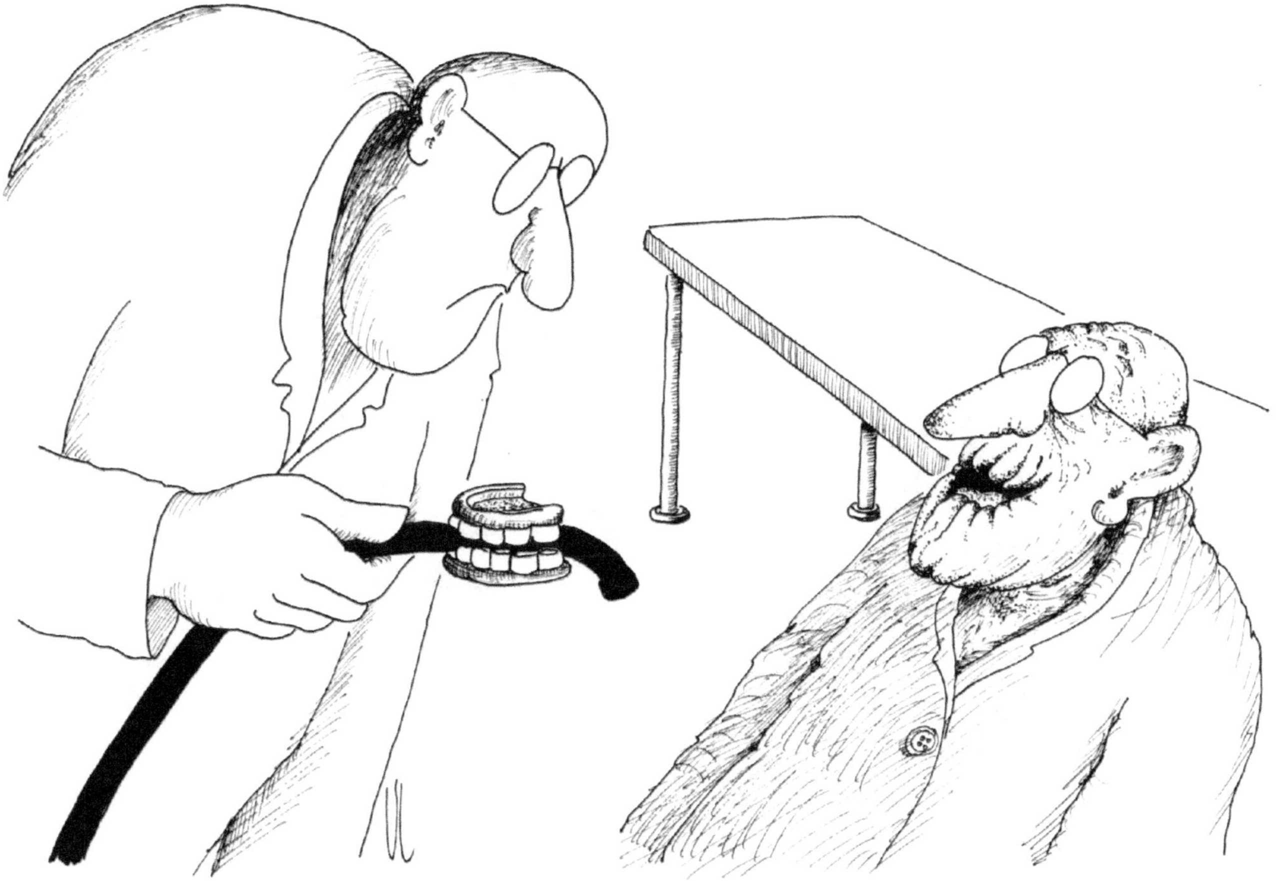

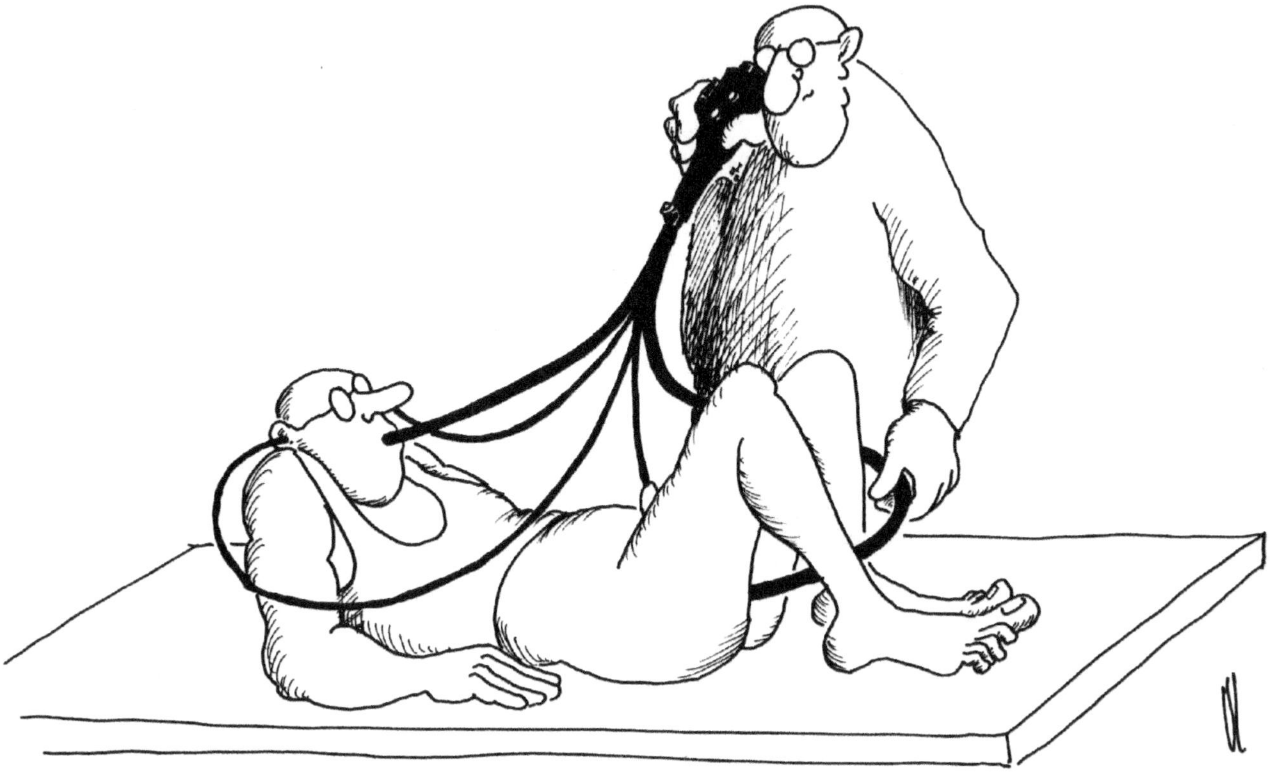

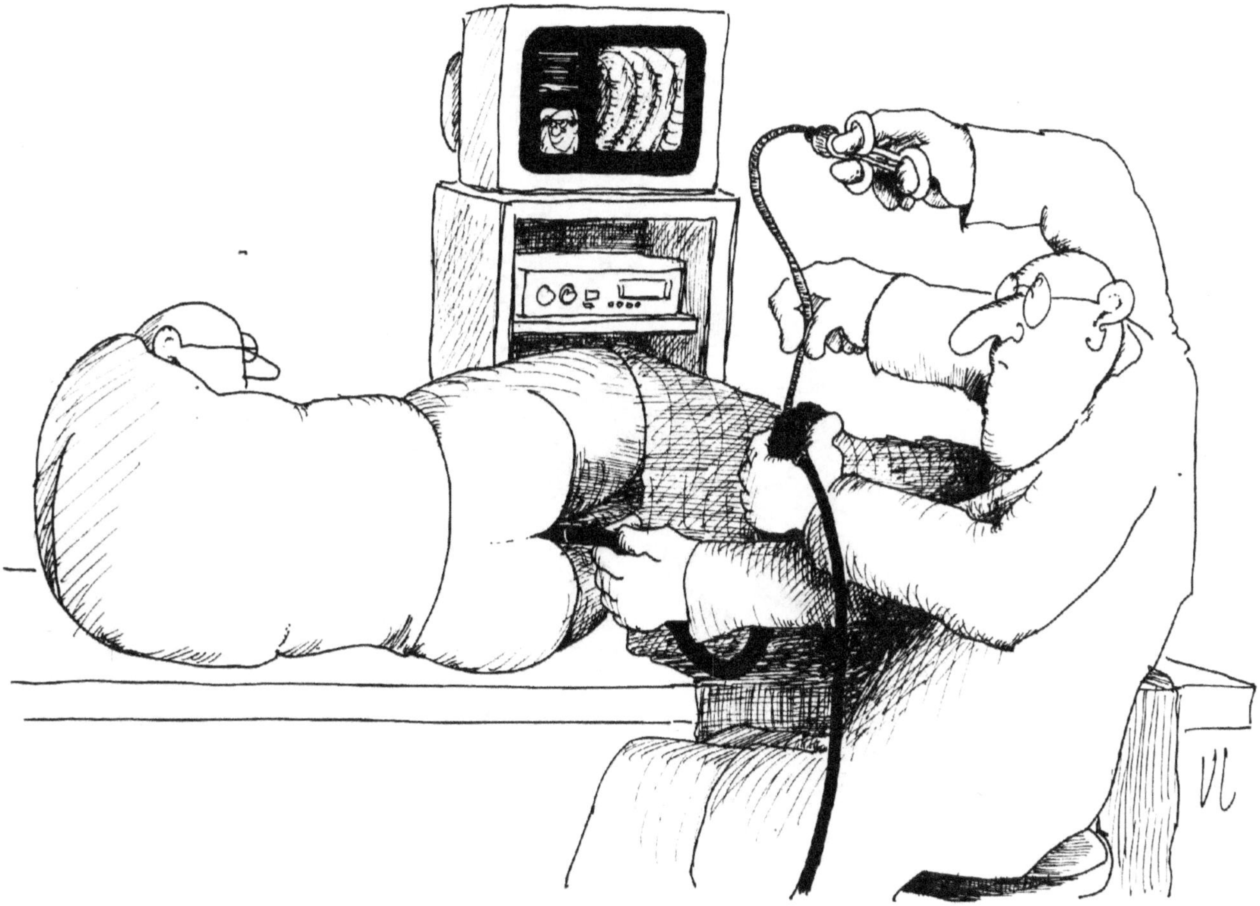

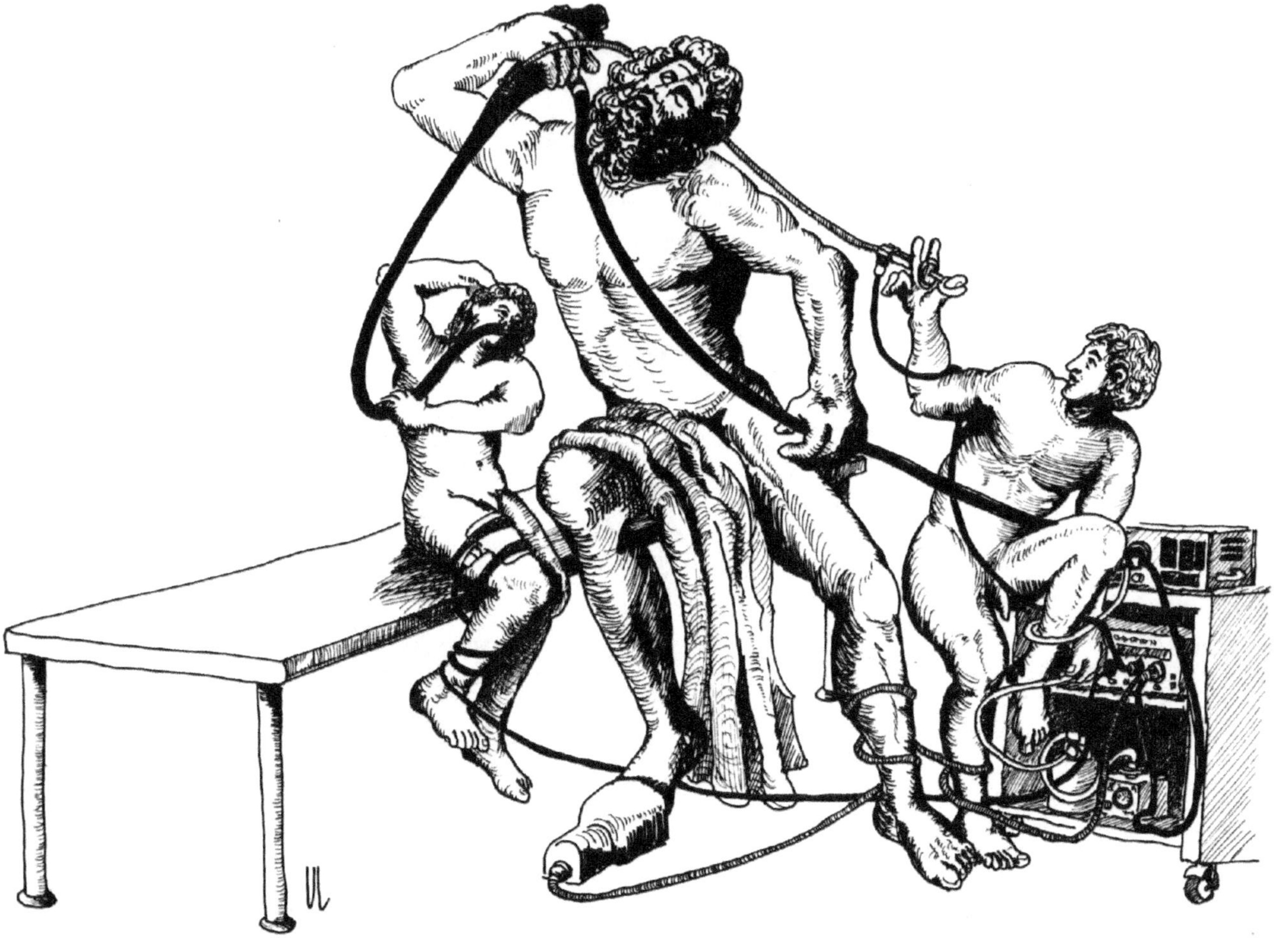

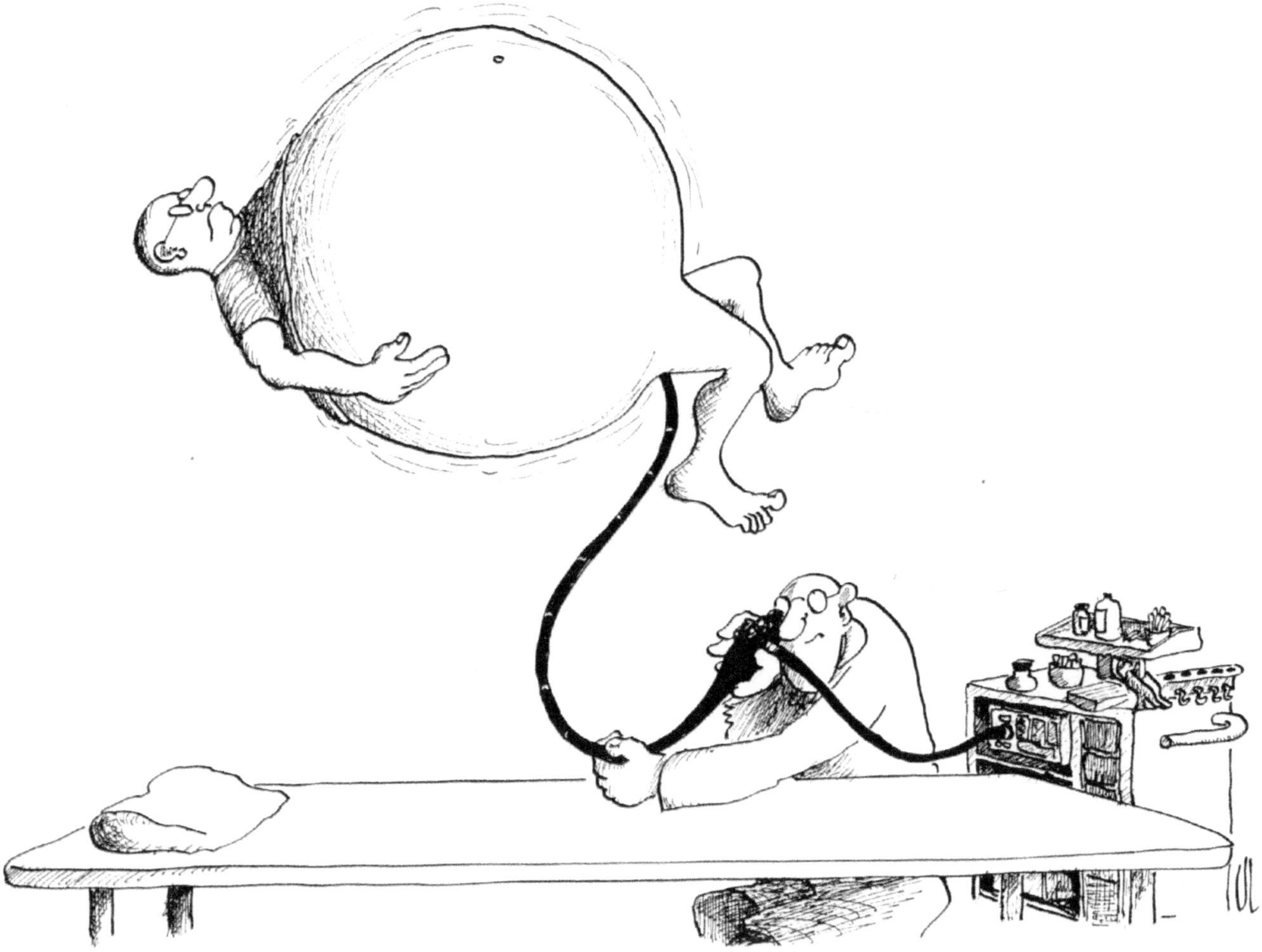

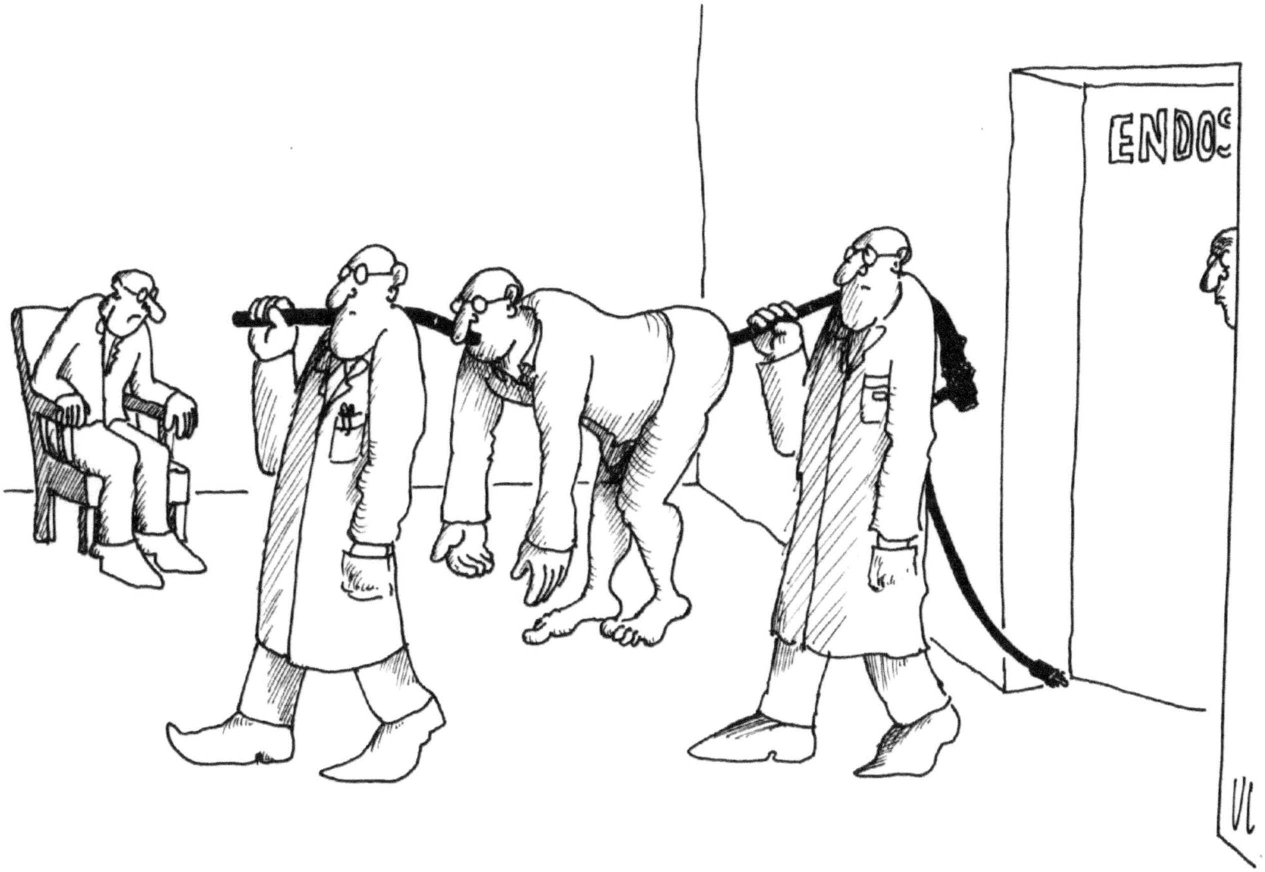
ENDOS

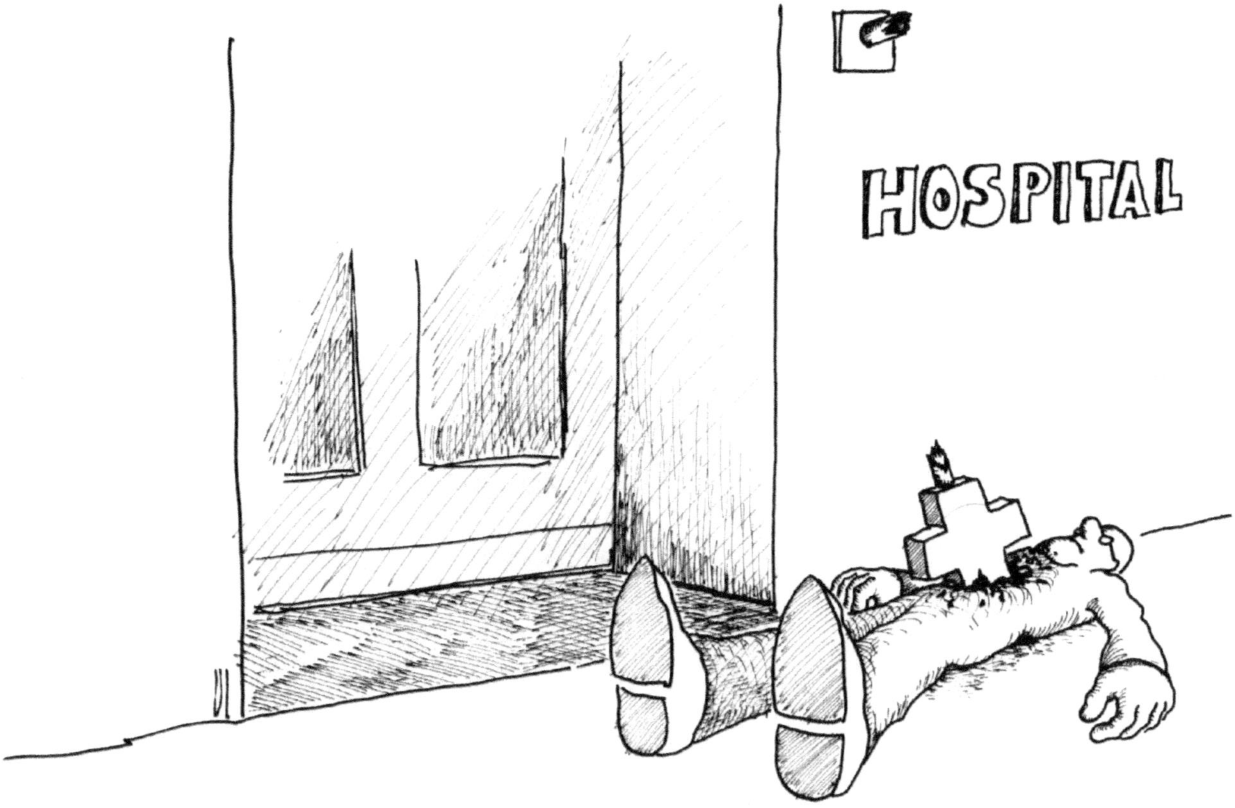
HOSPITAL

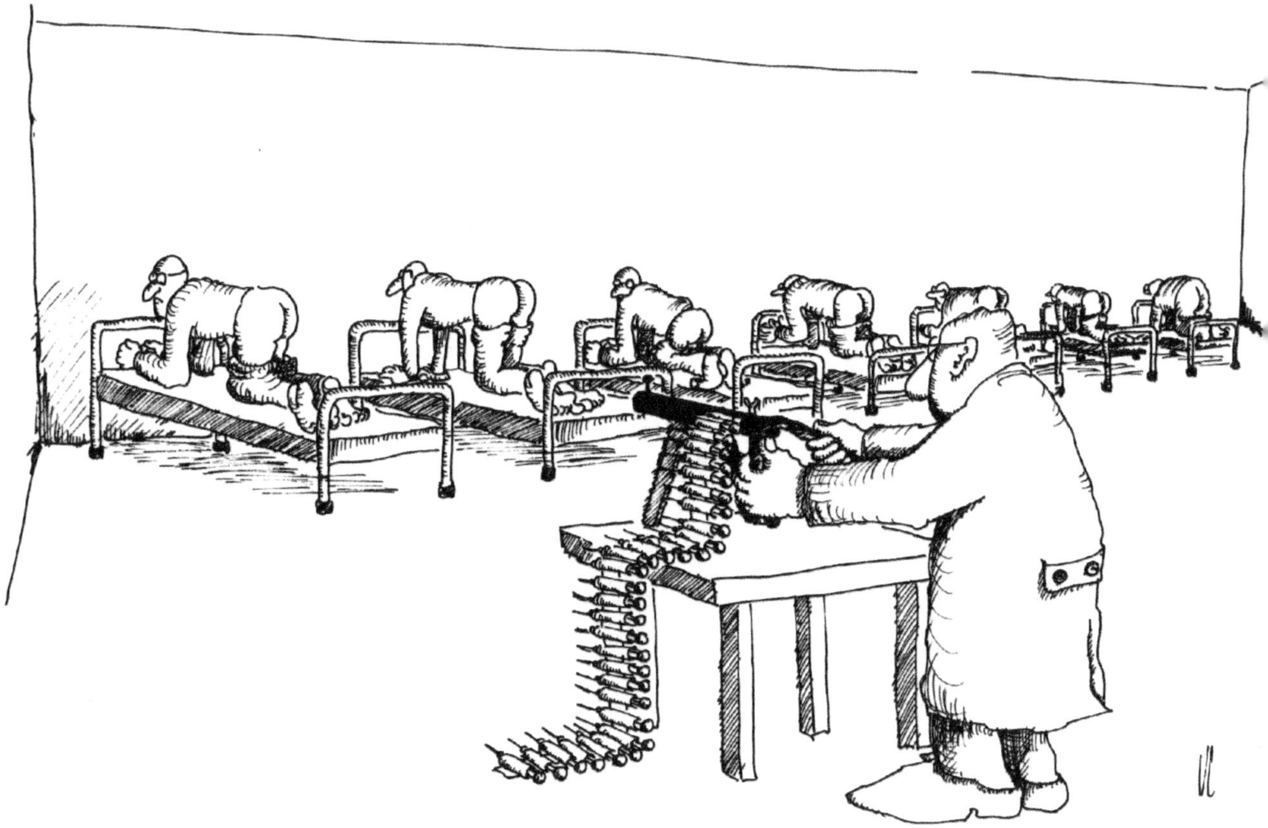

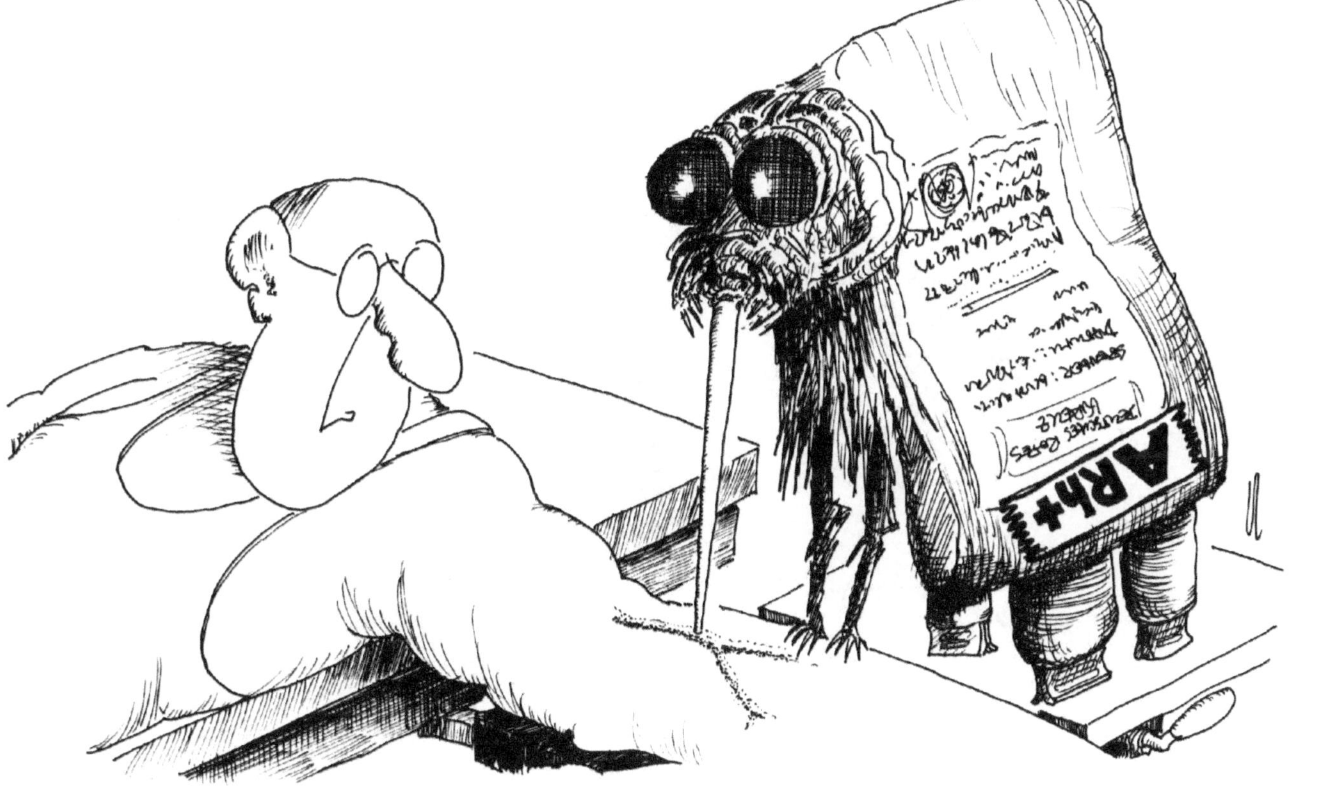
ARh+

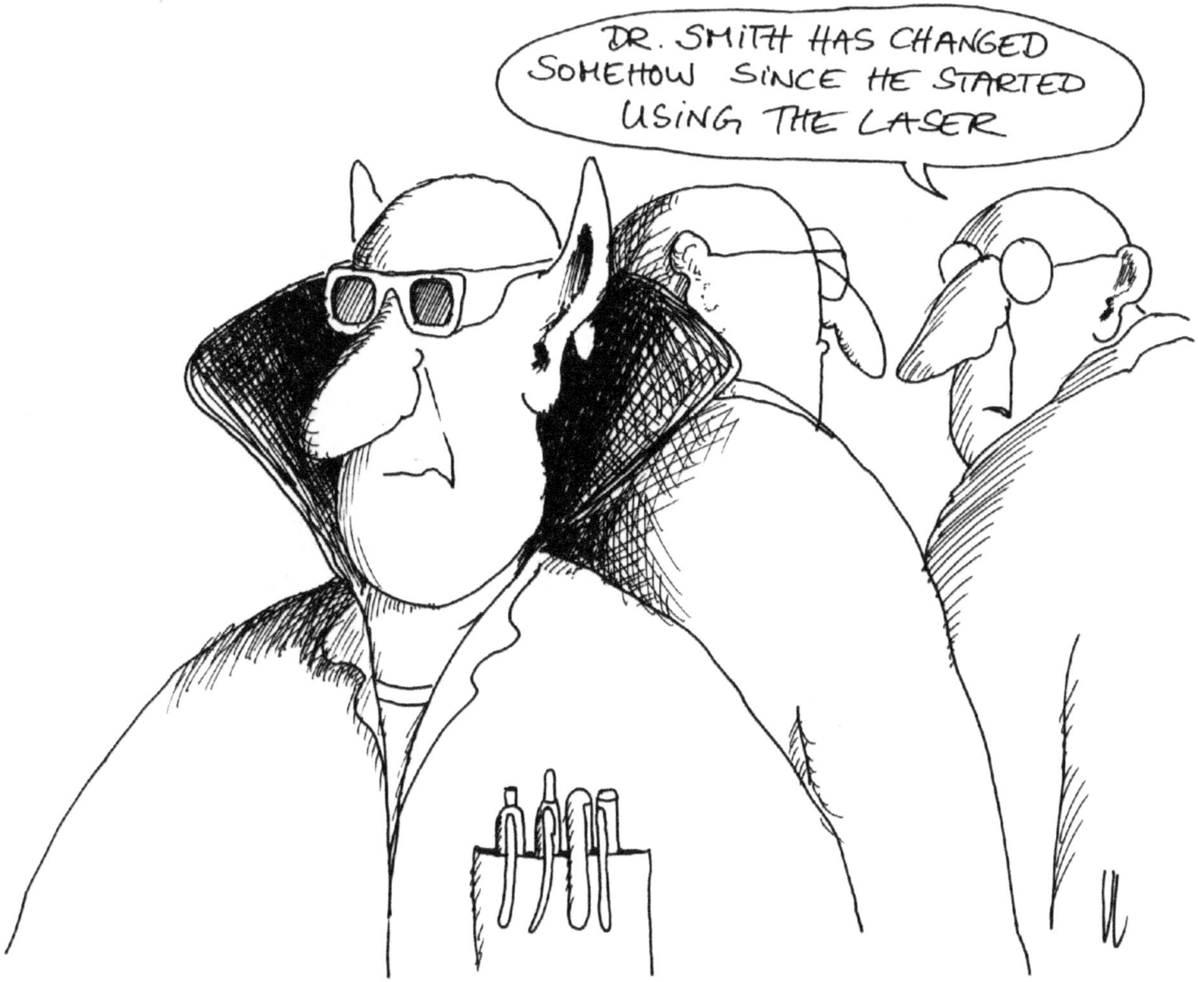
DR. SMITH HAS CHANGED SOMEHOW SINCE HE STARTED USING THE LASER

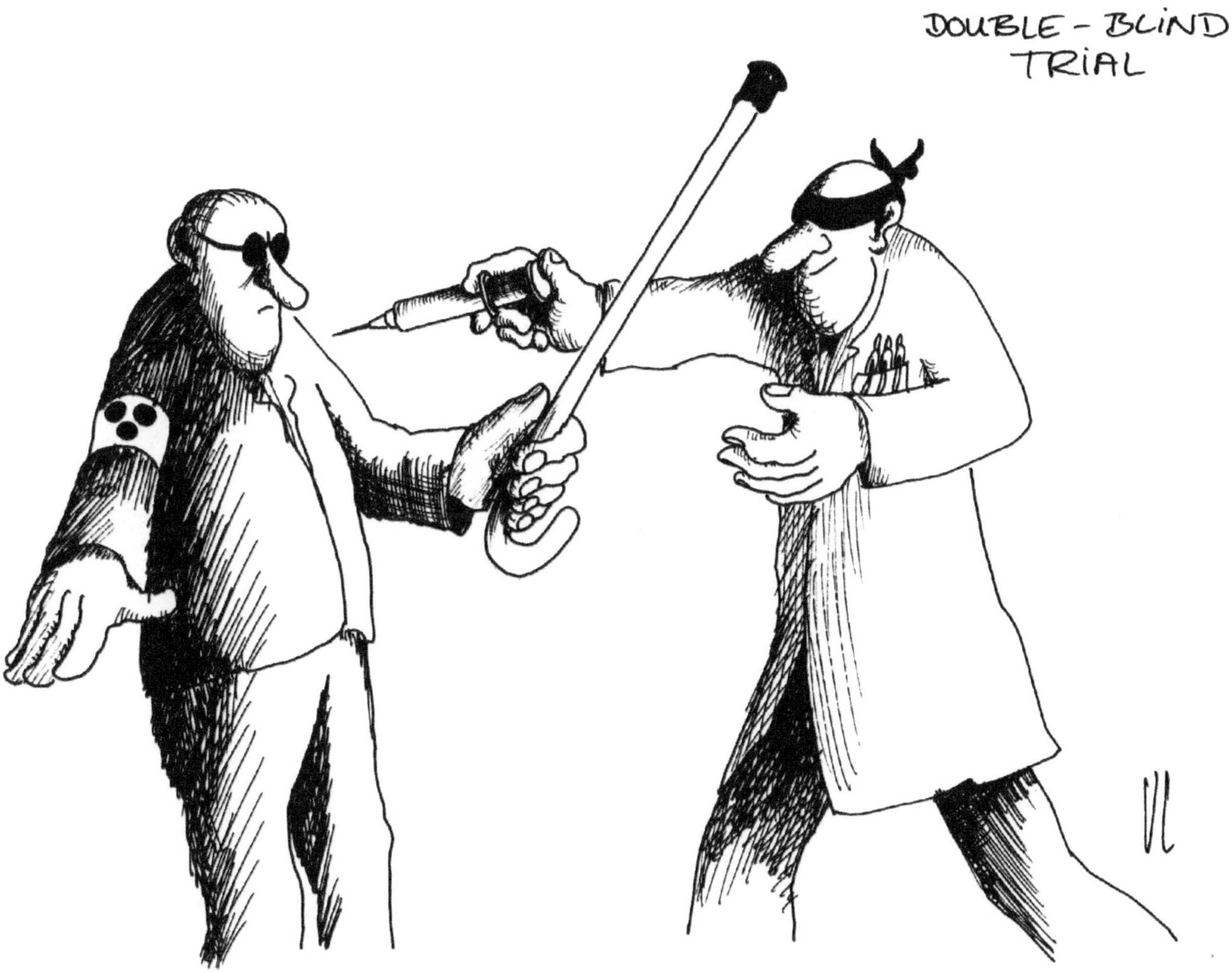
DOUBLE-BLIND
TRIAL

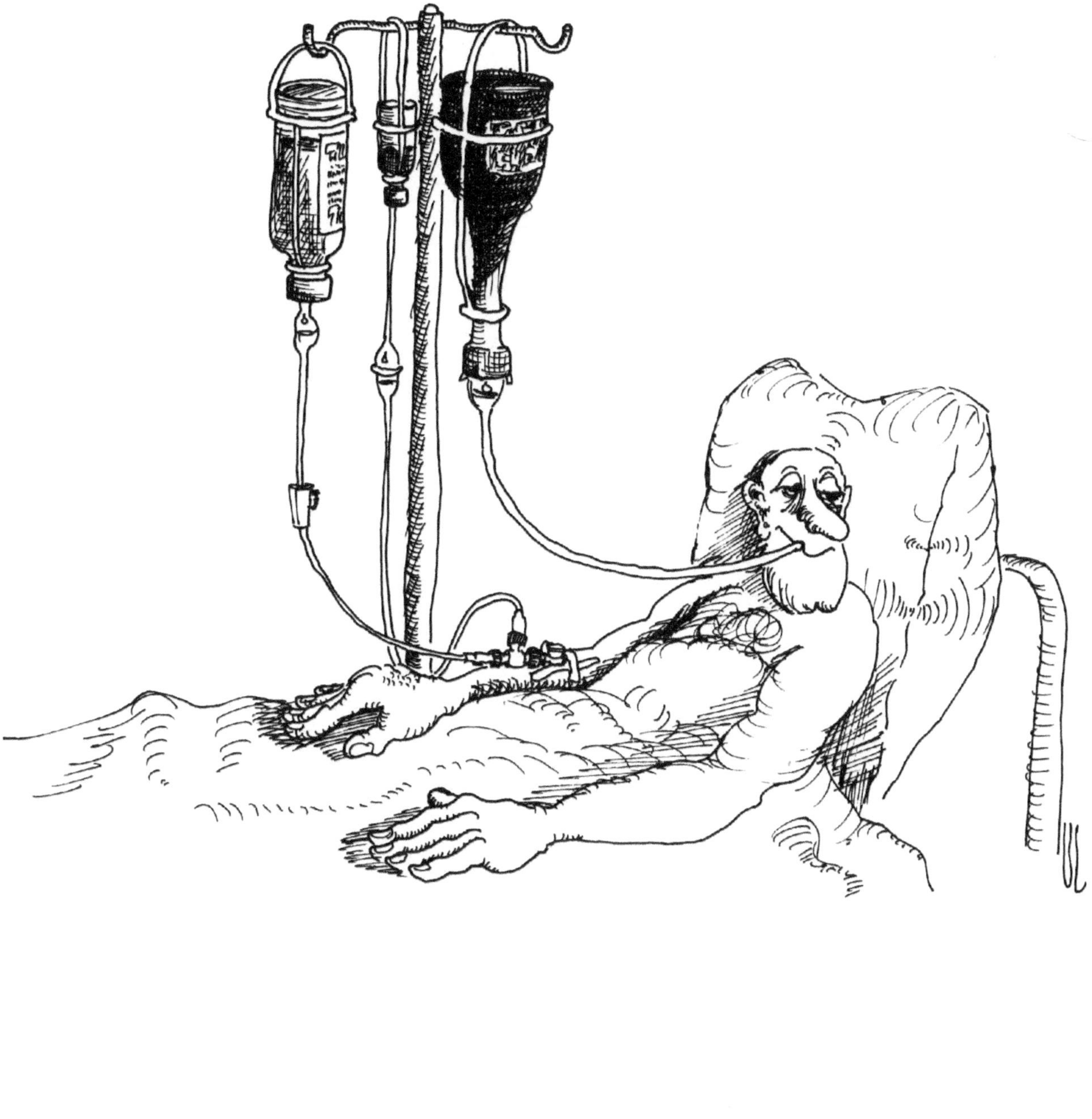

# ENT

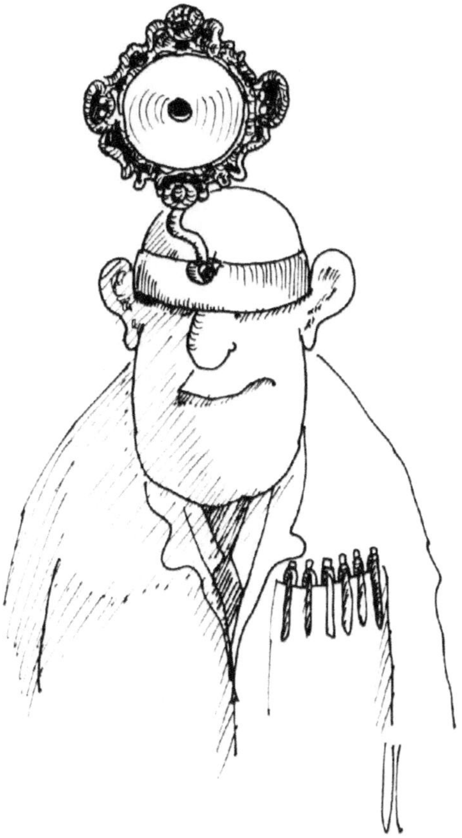

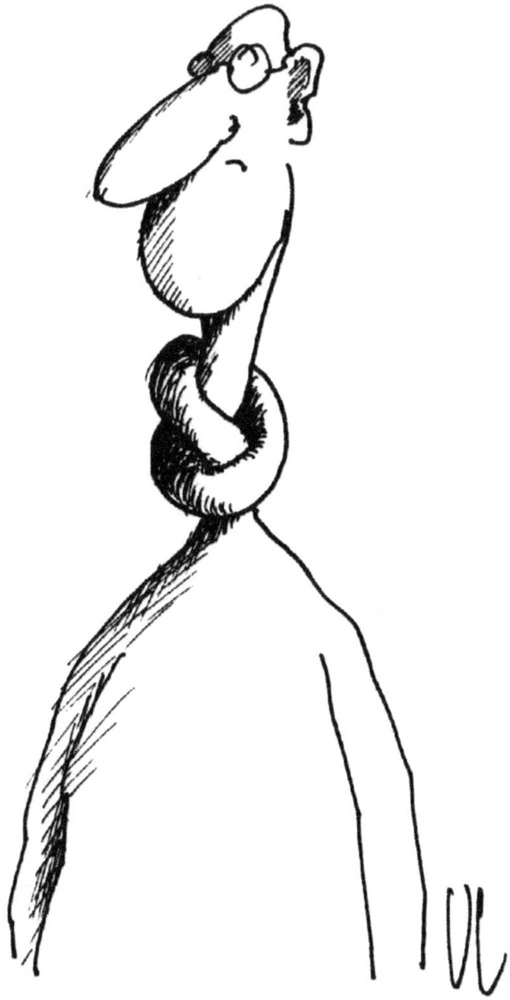

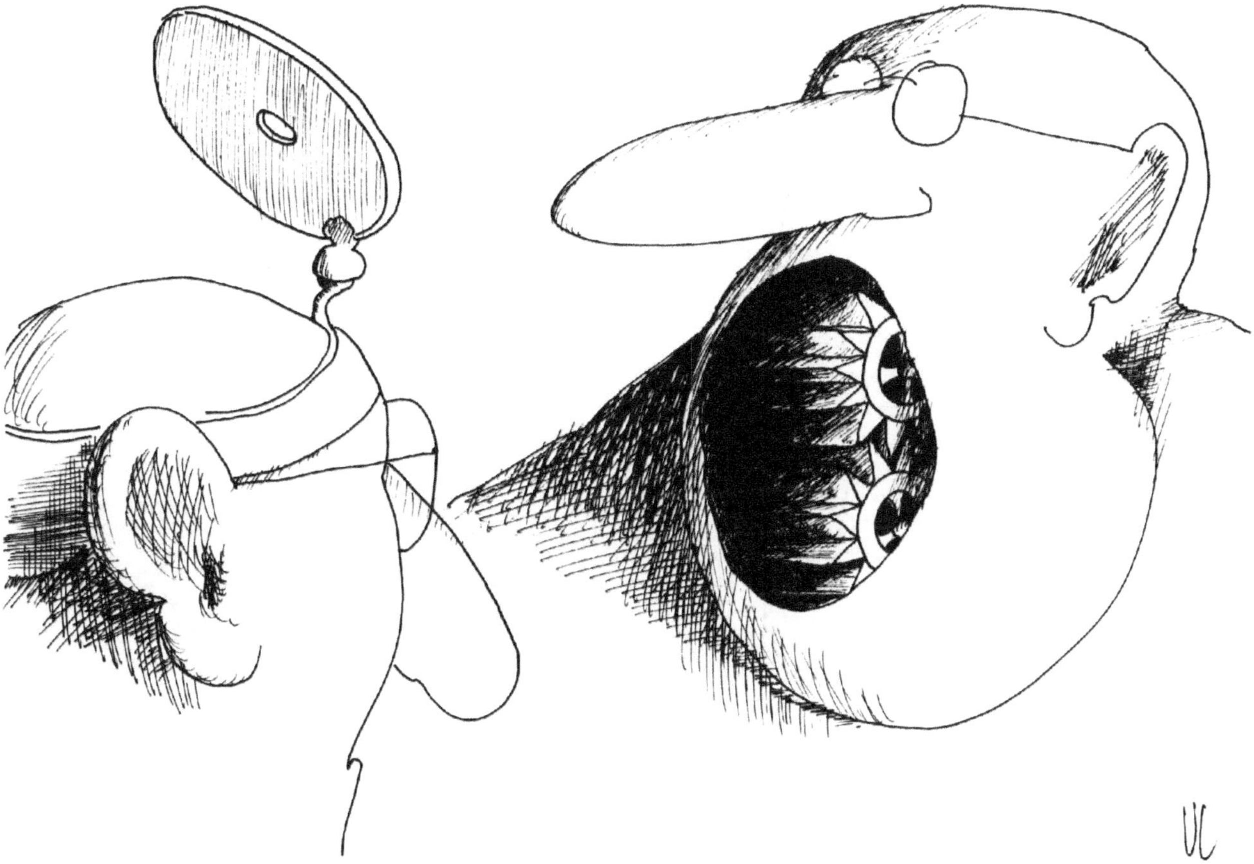

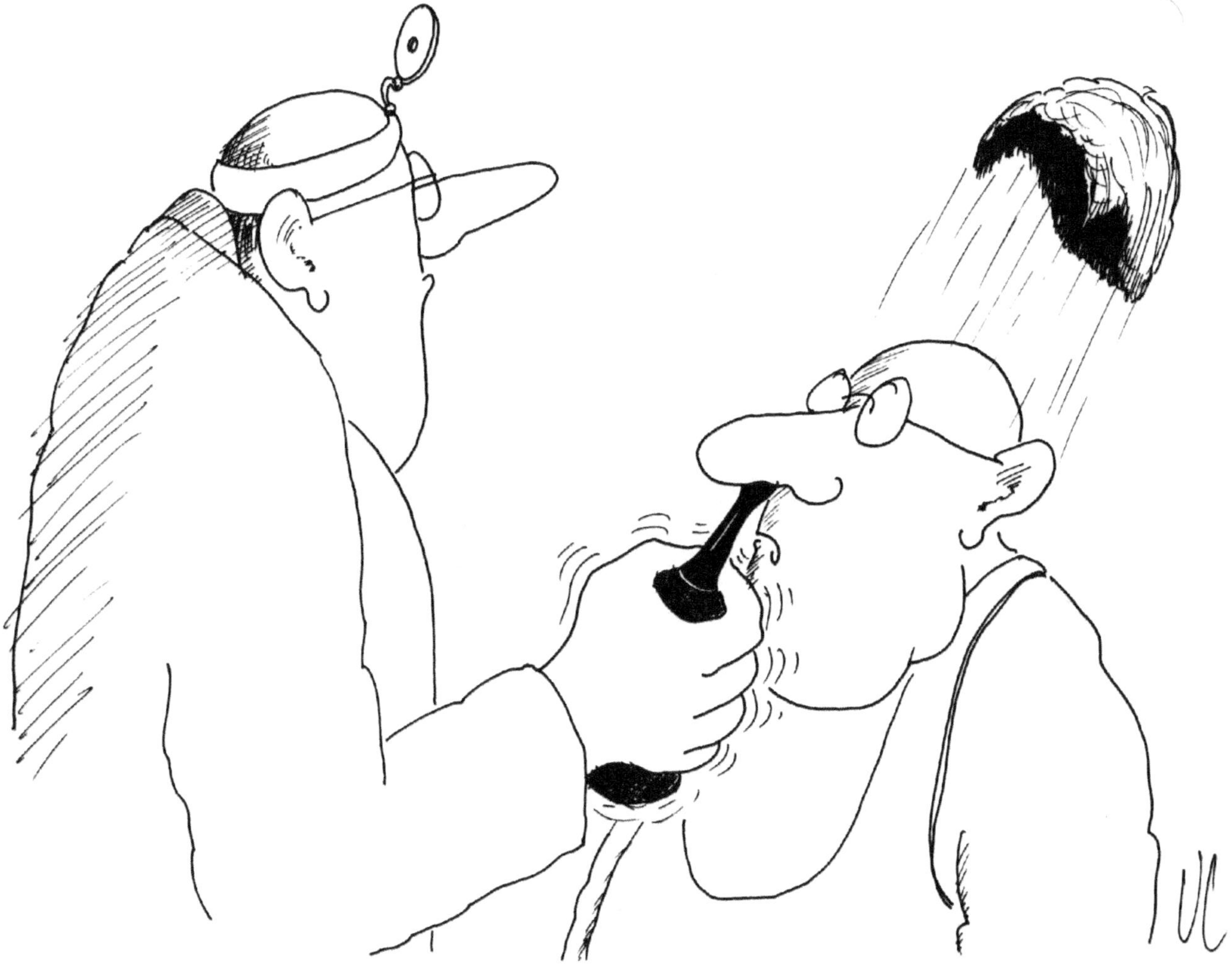

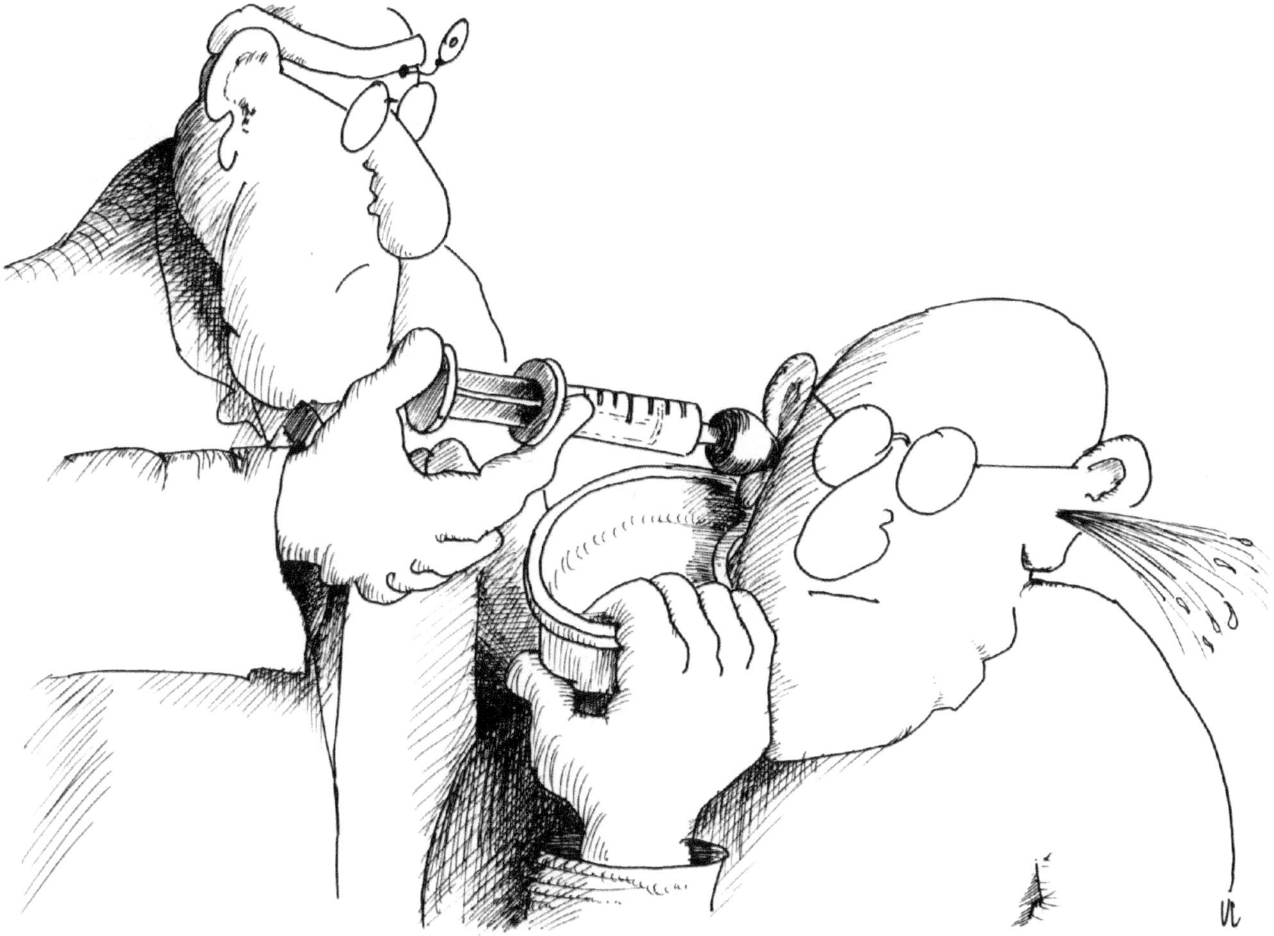

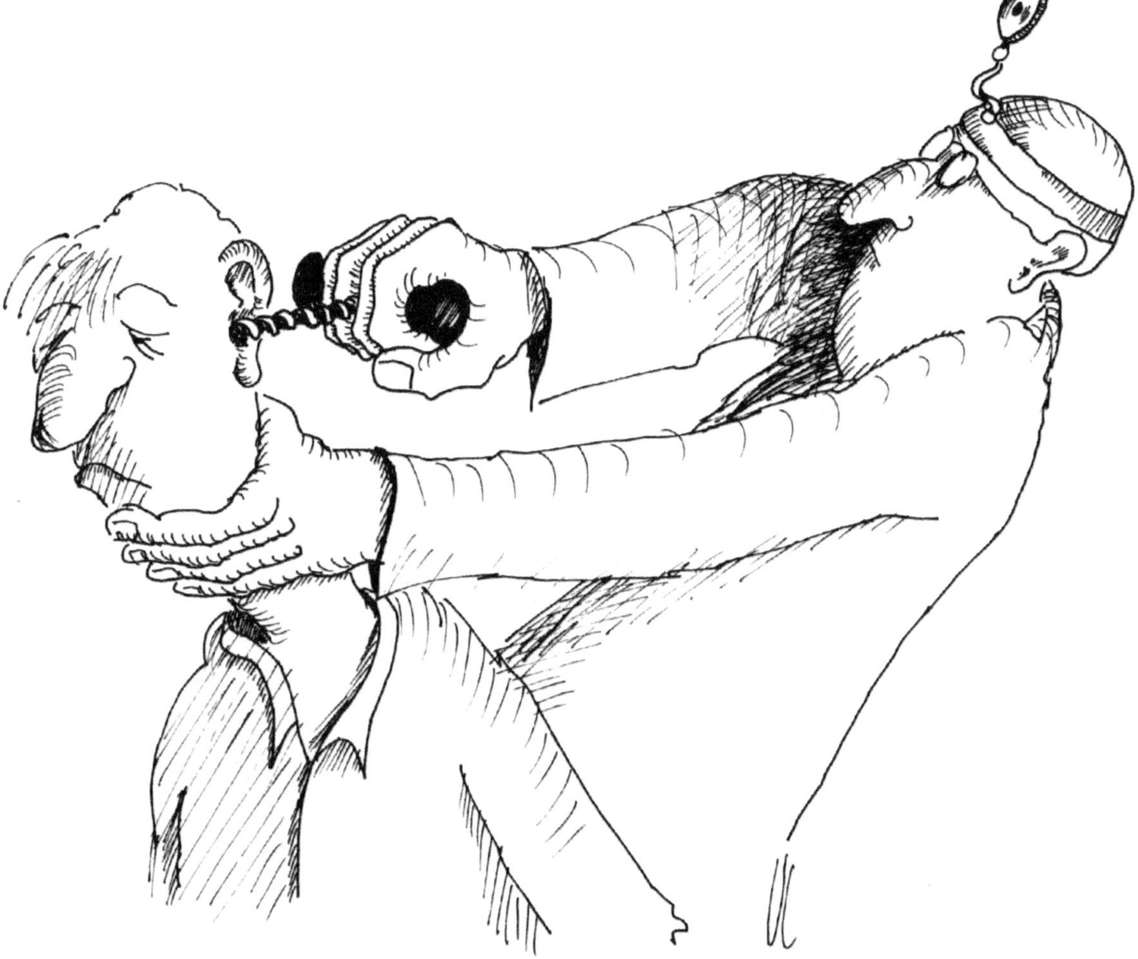

# INTERNAL MEDICINE

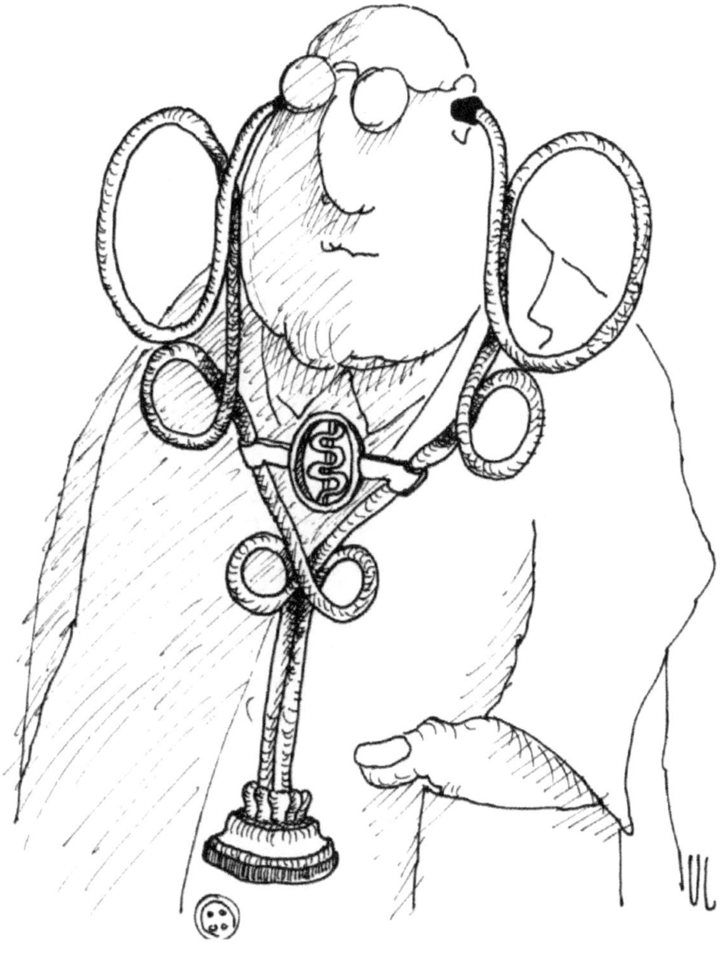

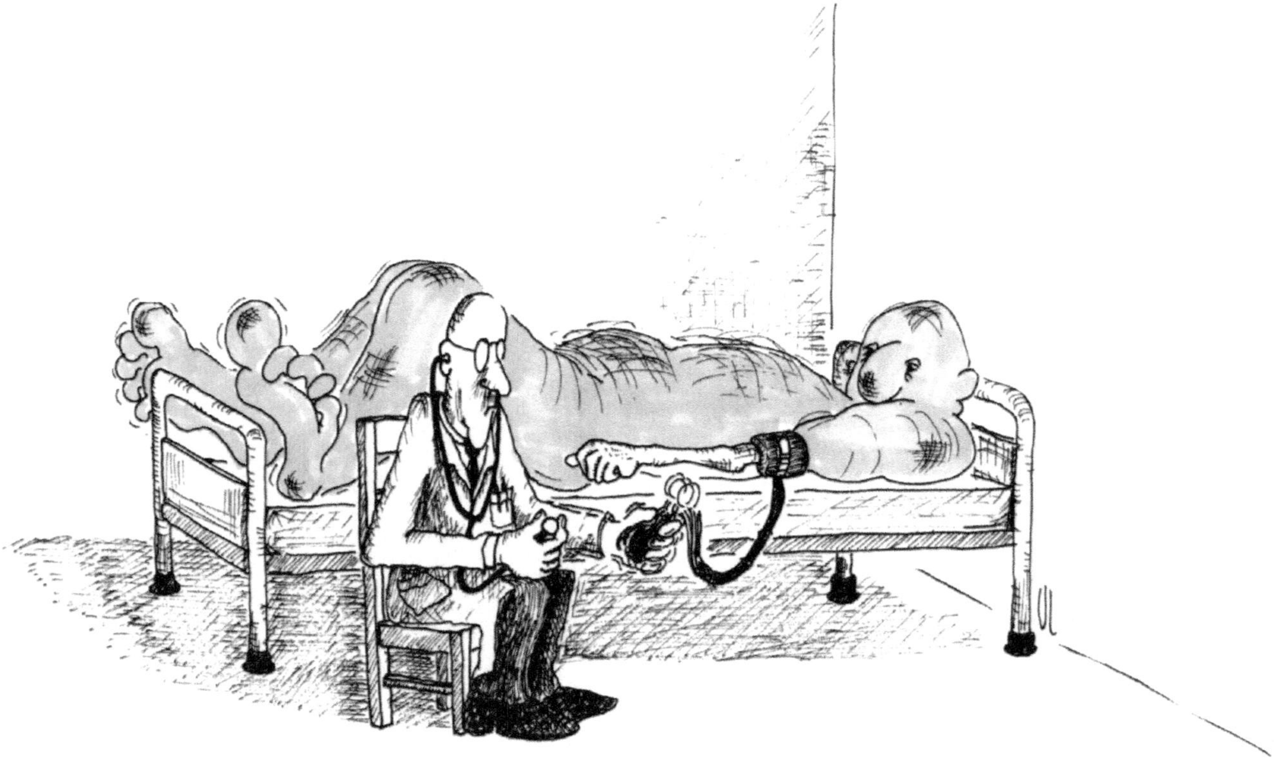

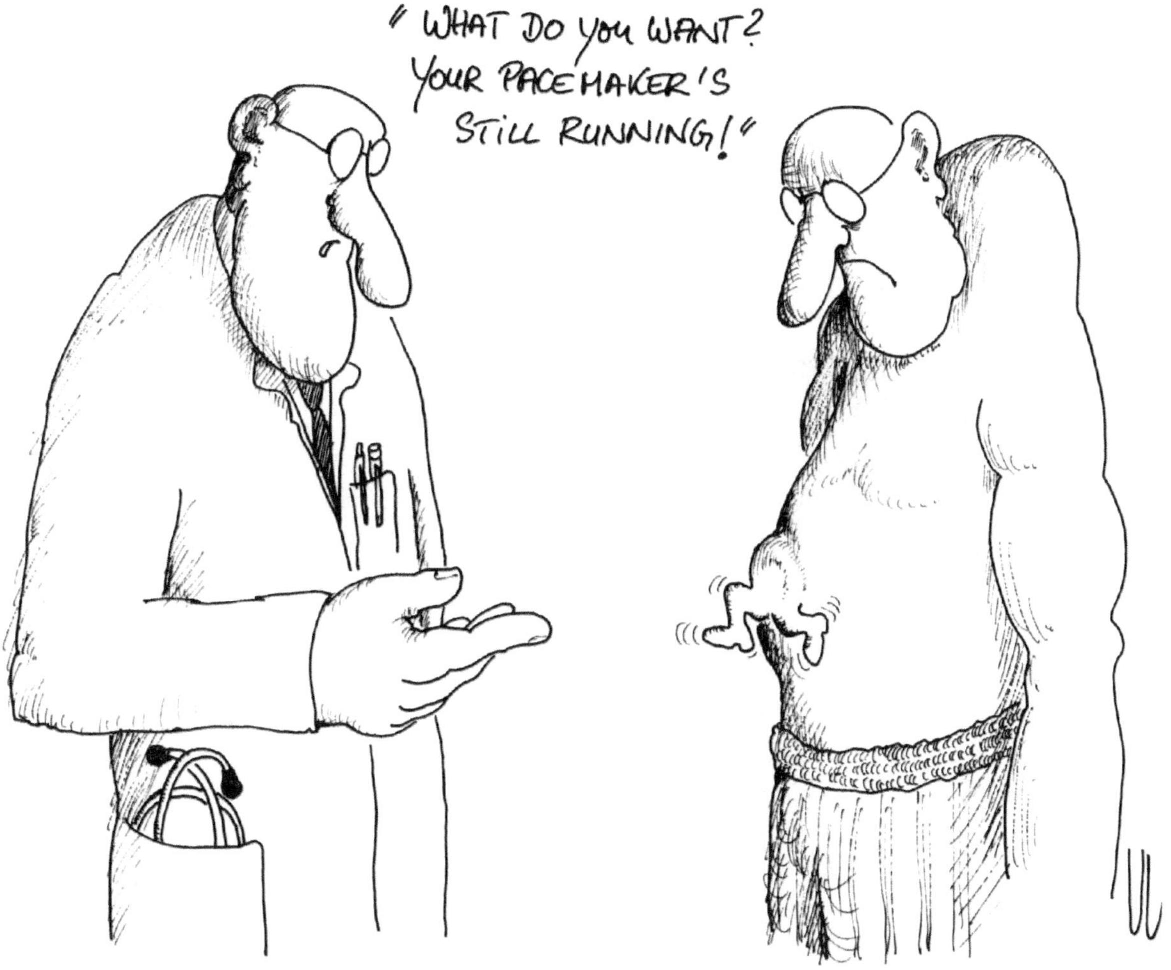
"WHAT DO YOU WANT?
YOUR PACEMAKER'S
STILL RUNNING!"

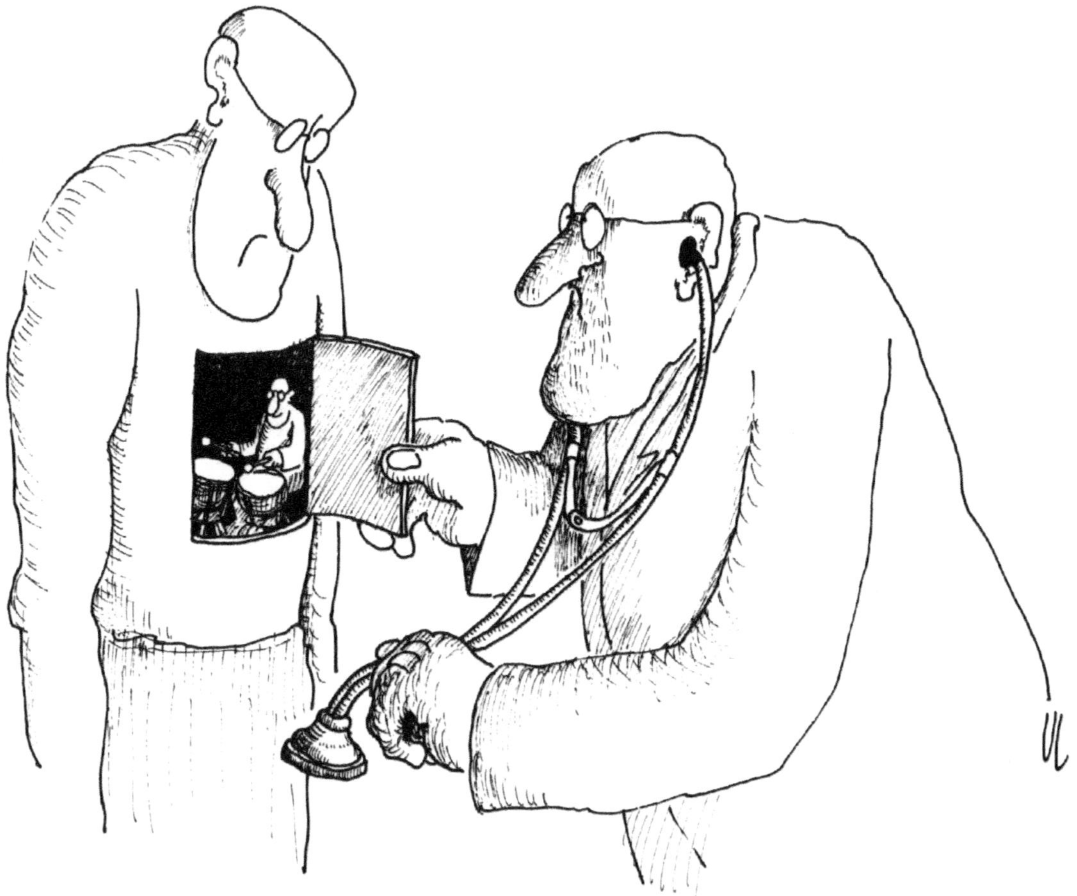

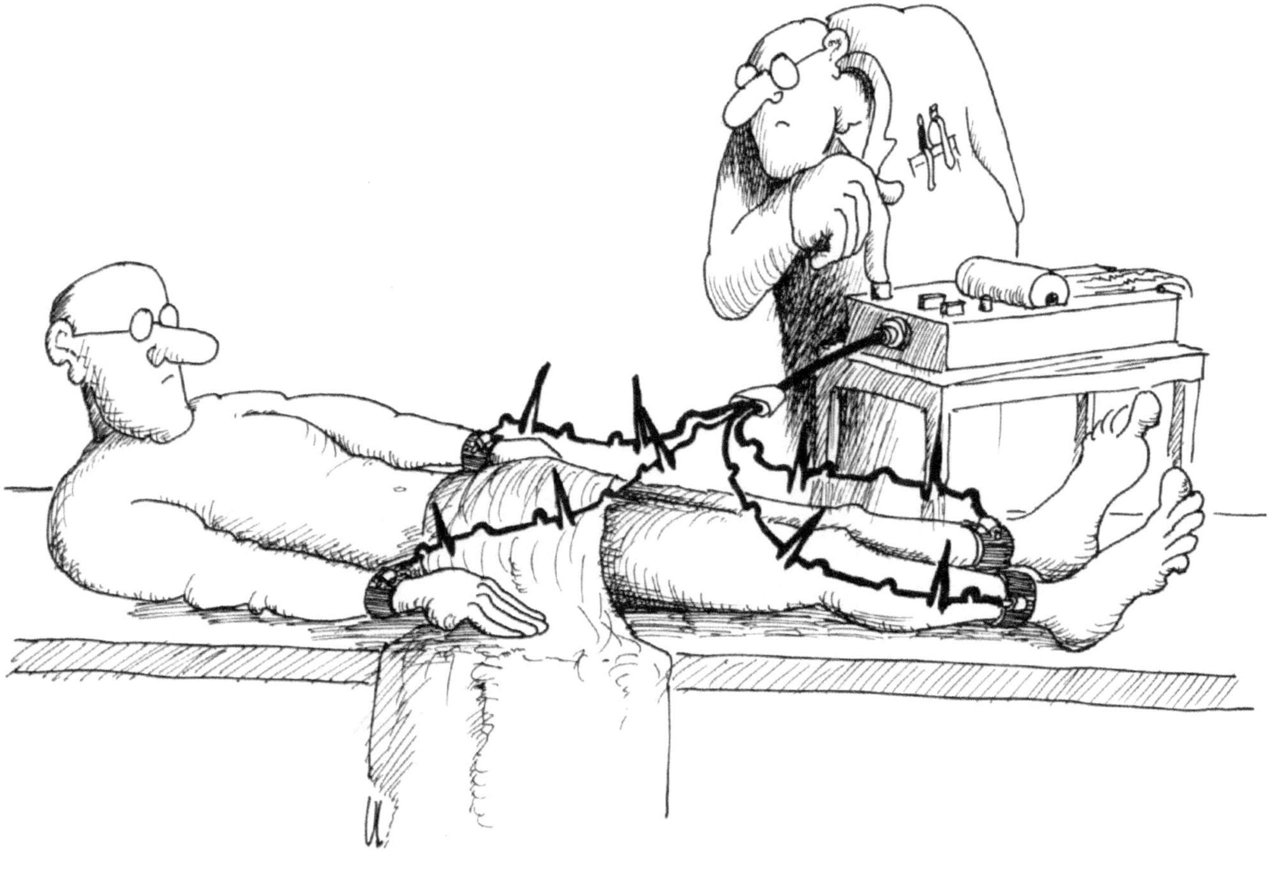

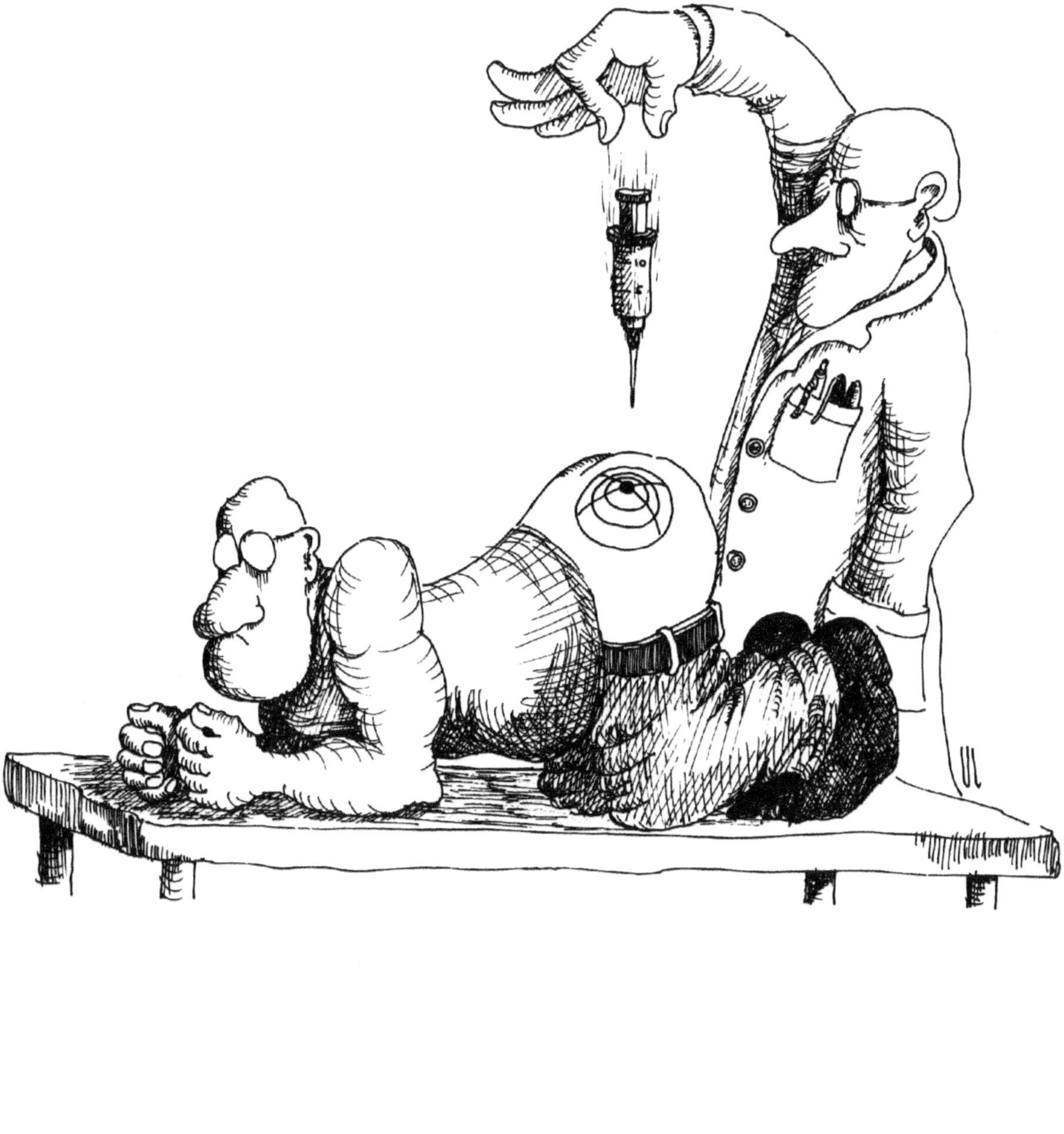

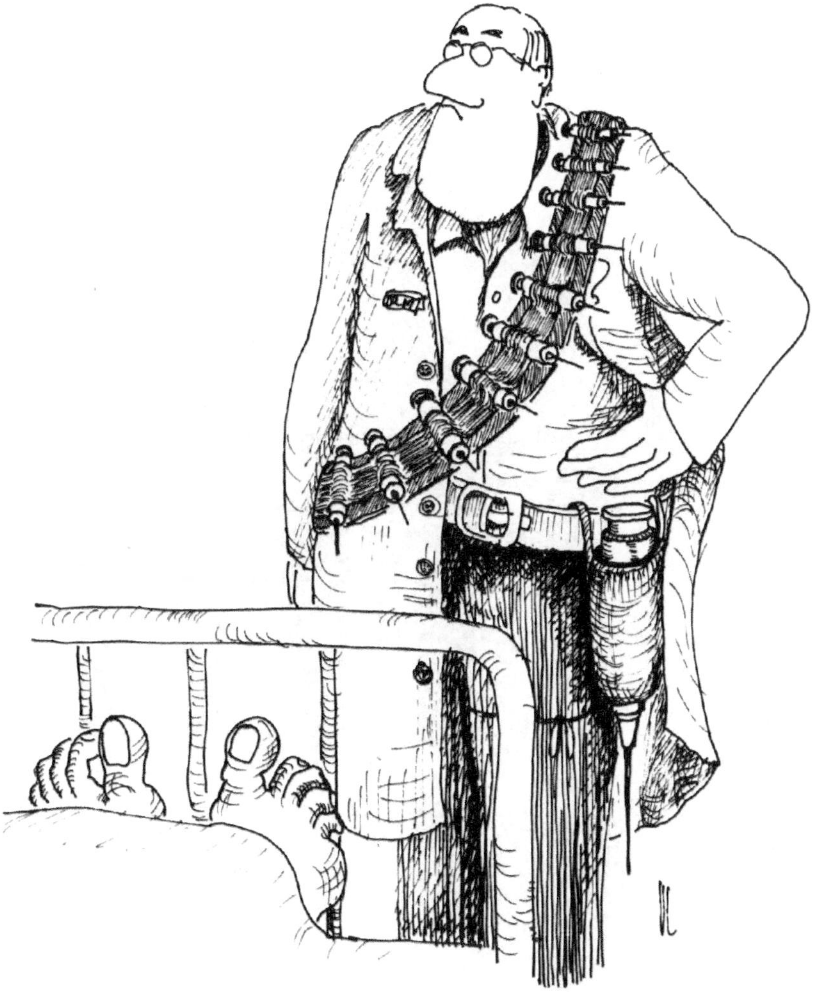

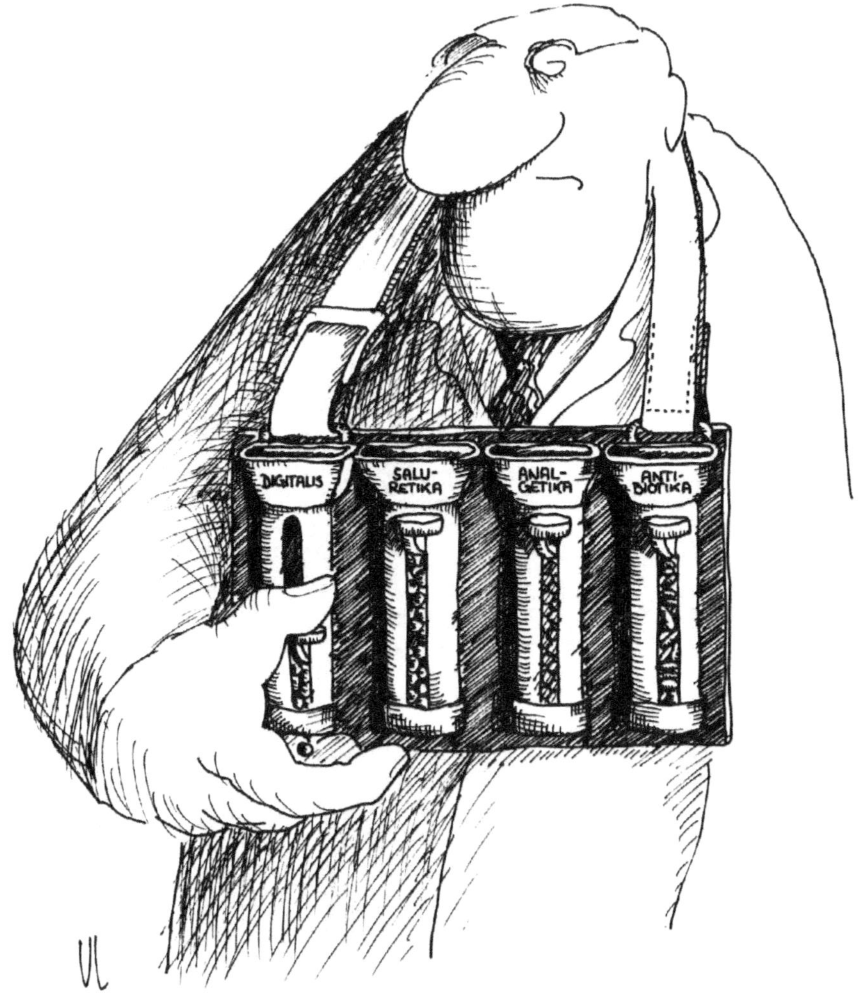
DIGITALIS
SALU-
RETIKA
ANAL-
GETIKA
ANTI-
BIOTIKA
UL

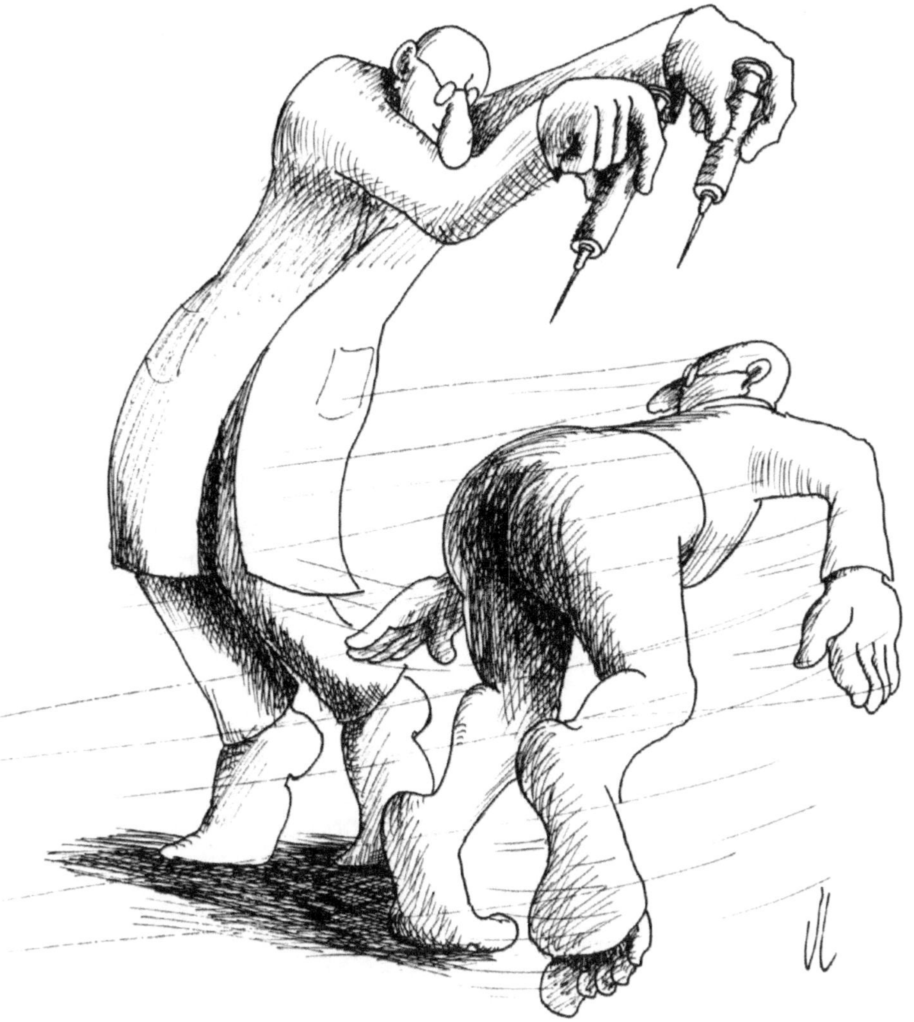

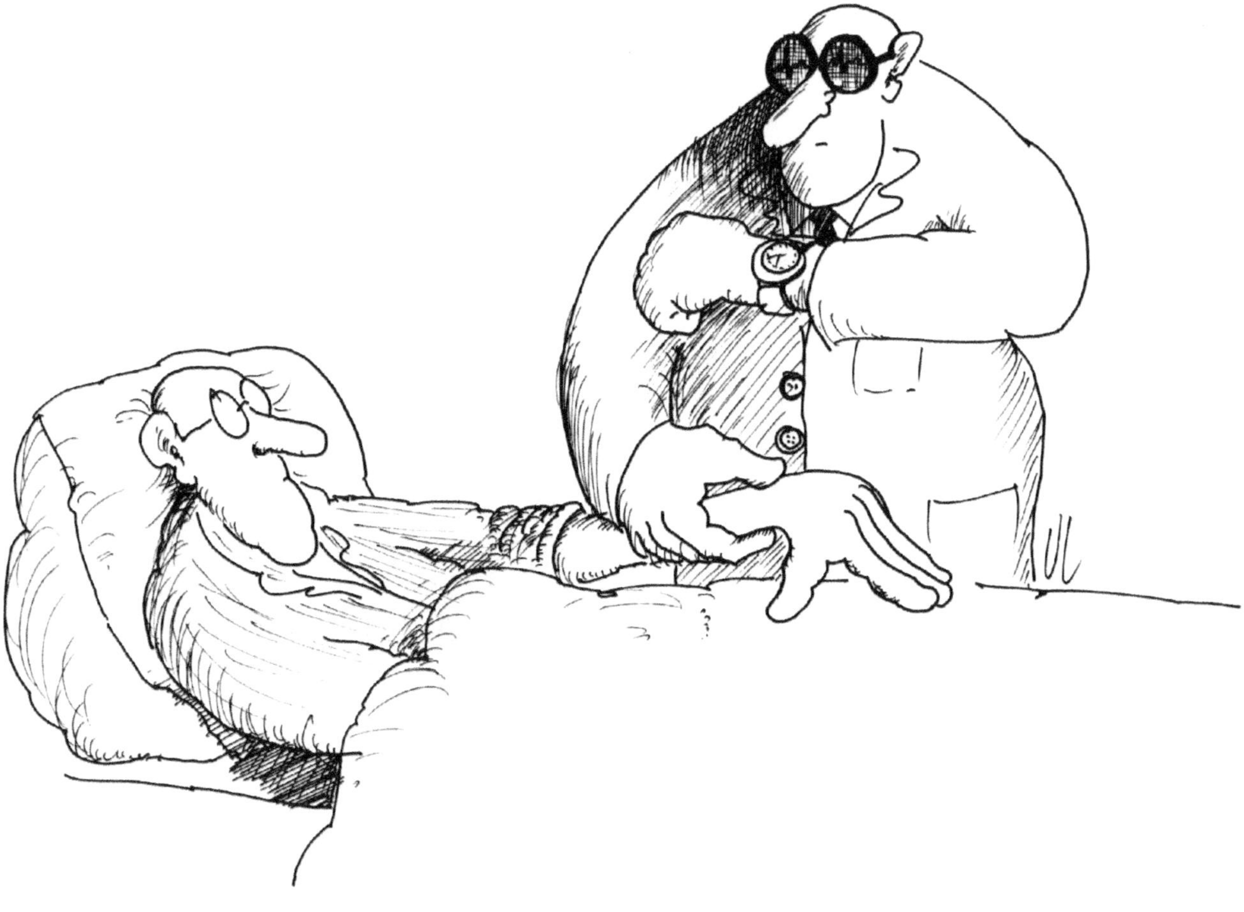

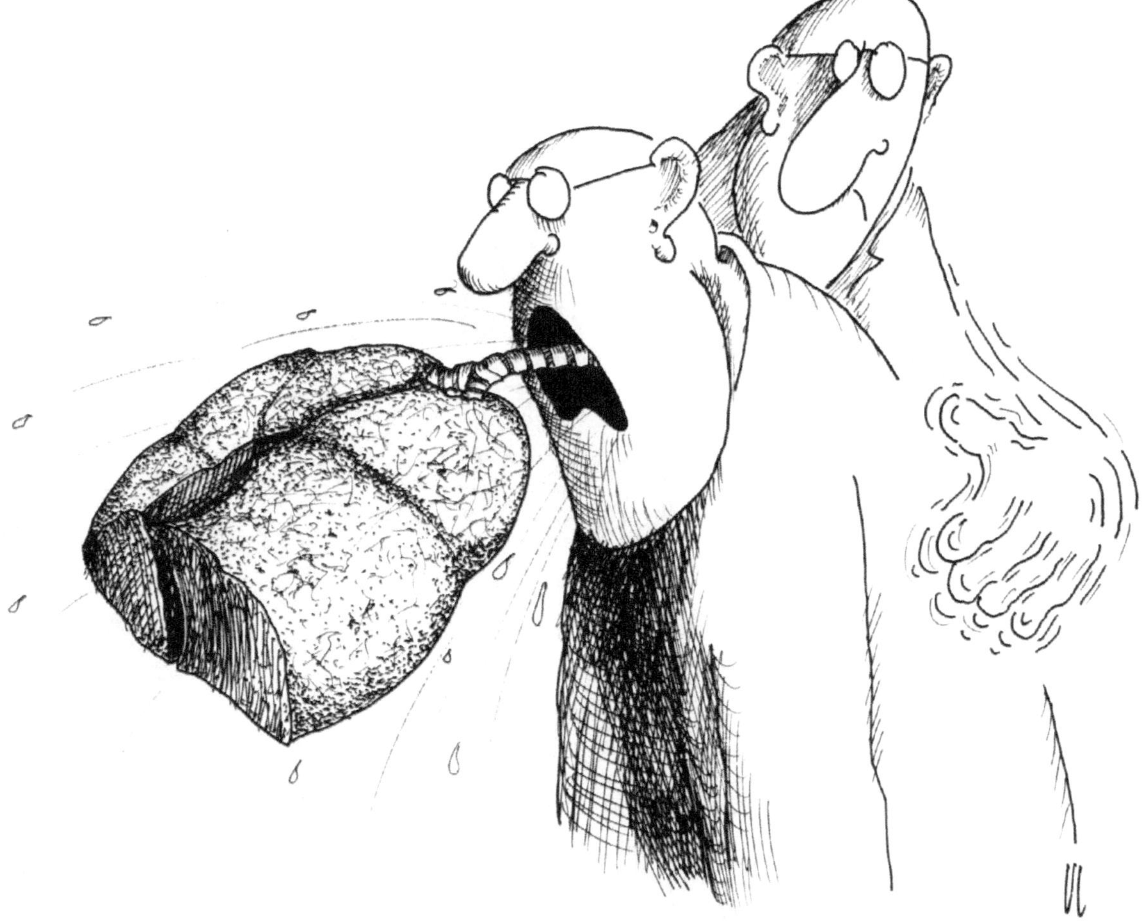

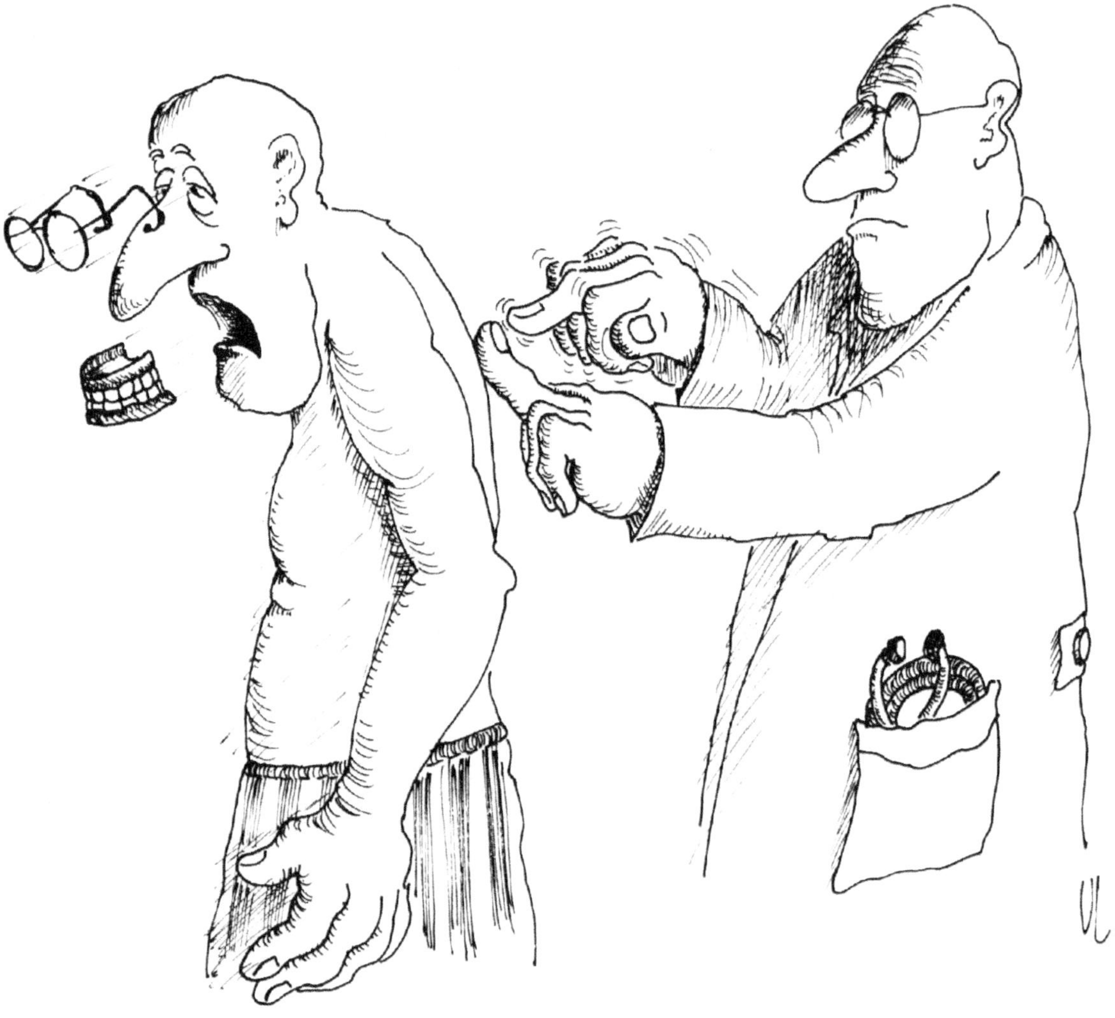

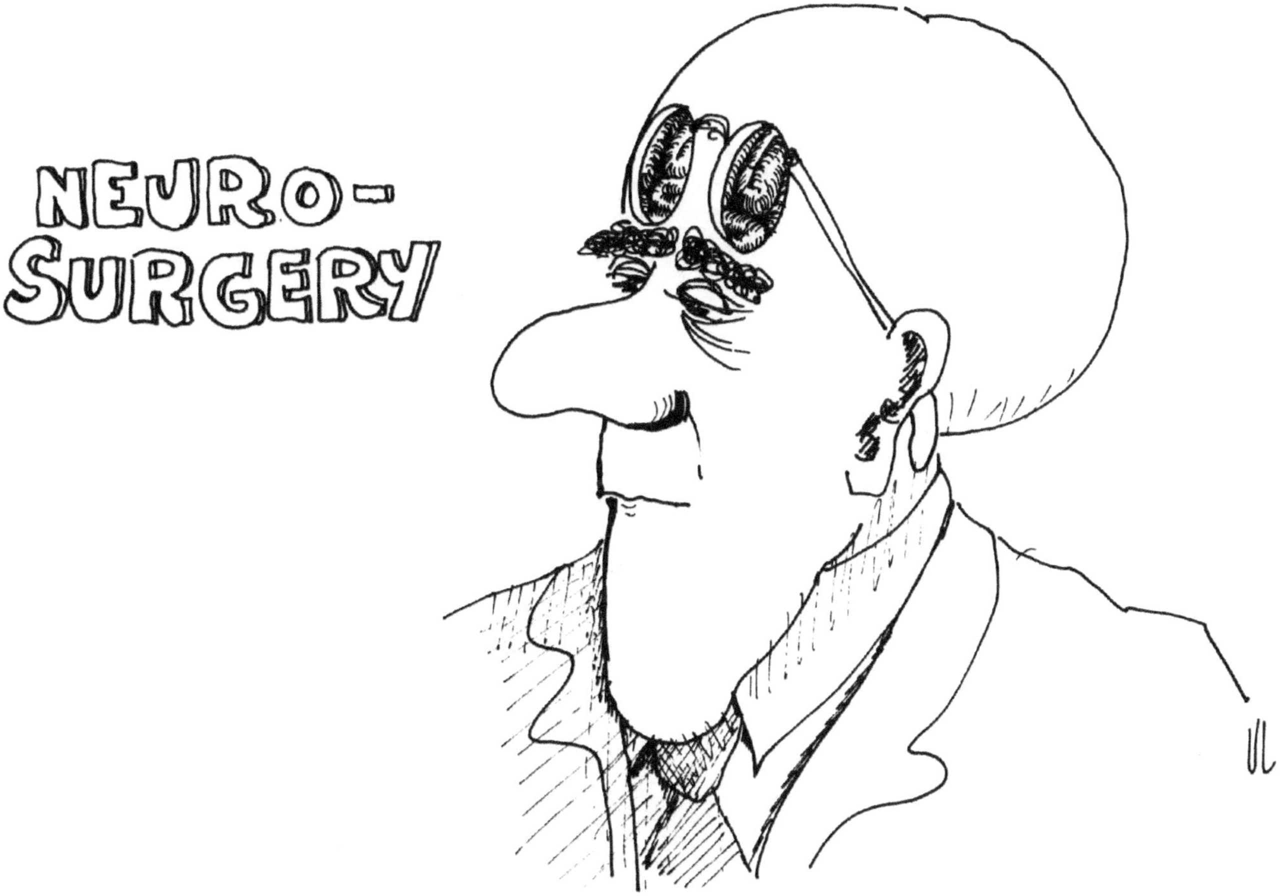
NEURO-
SURGERY

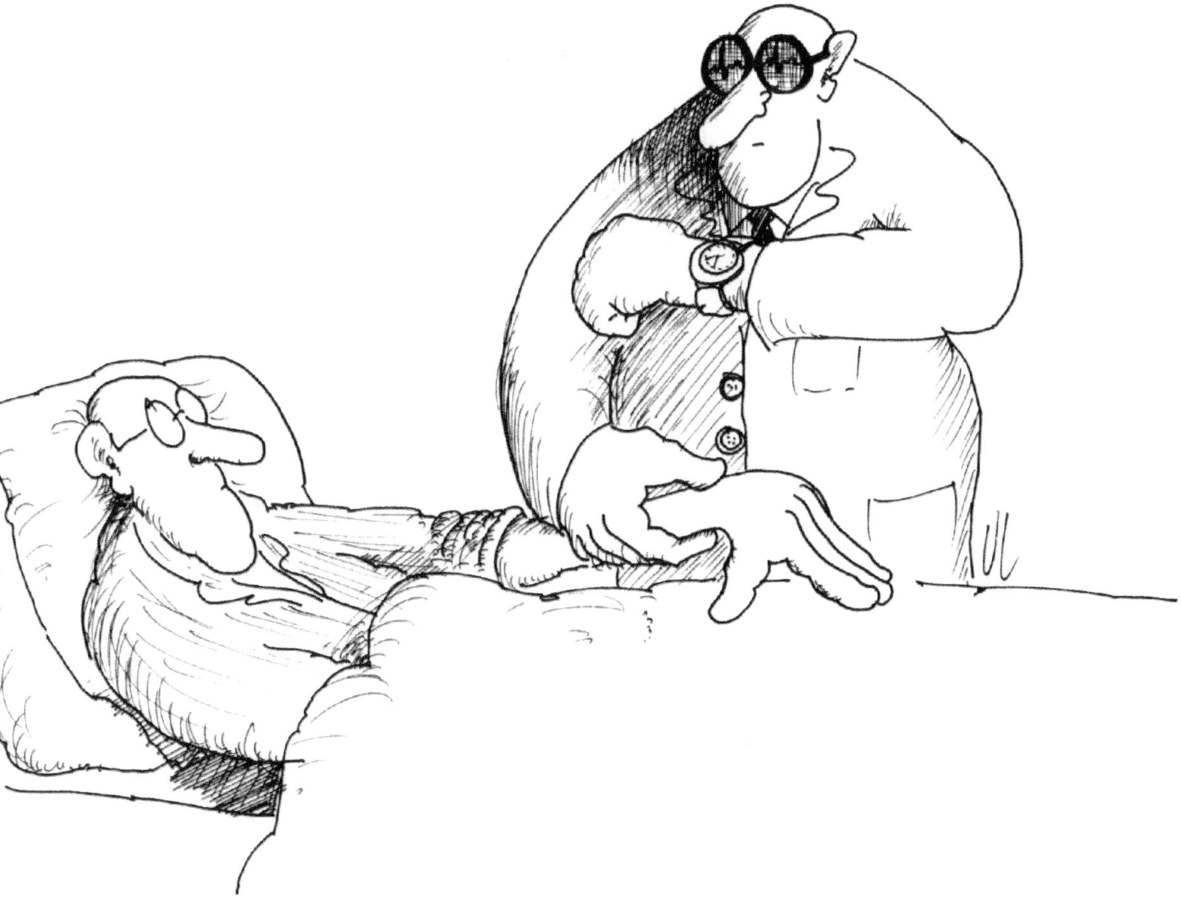

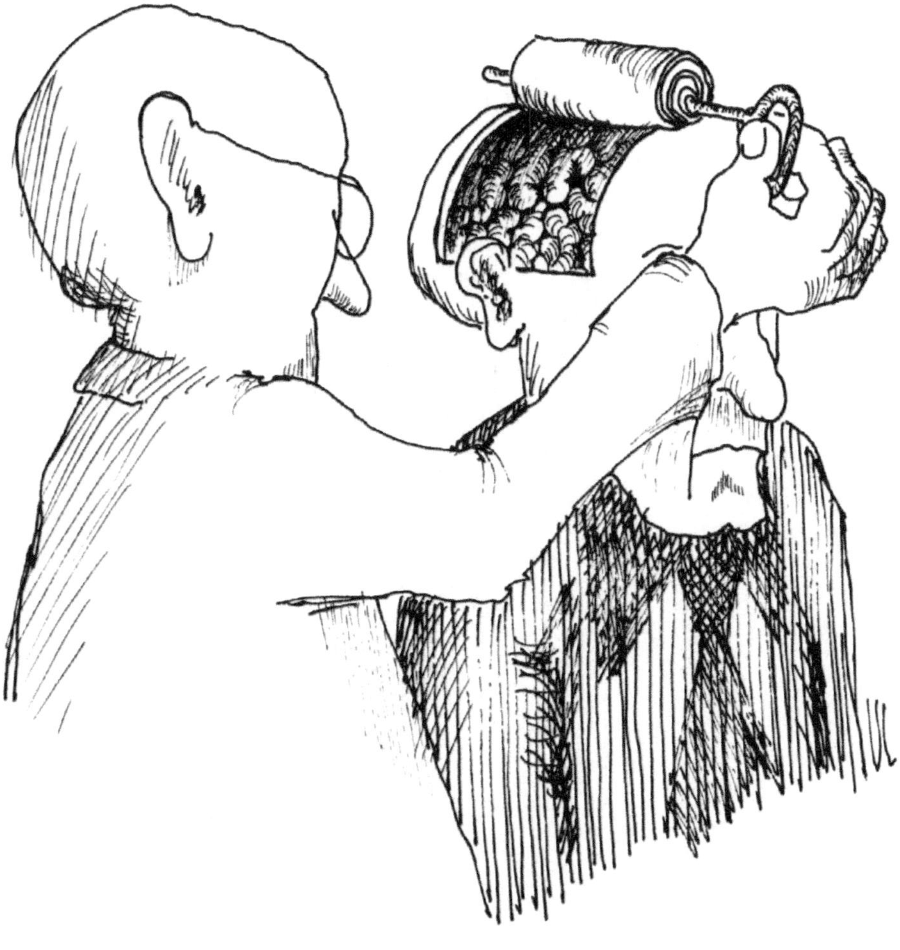

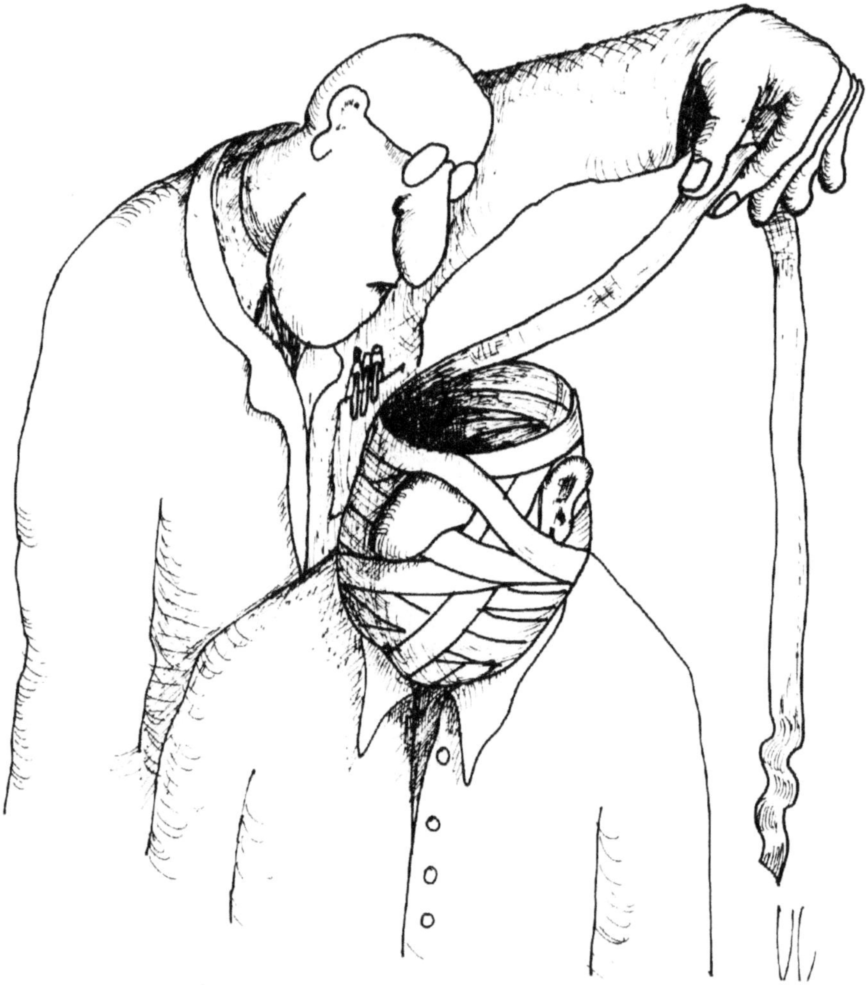

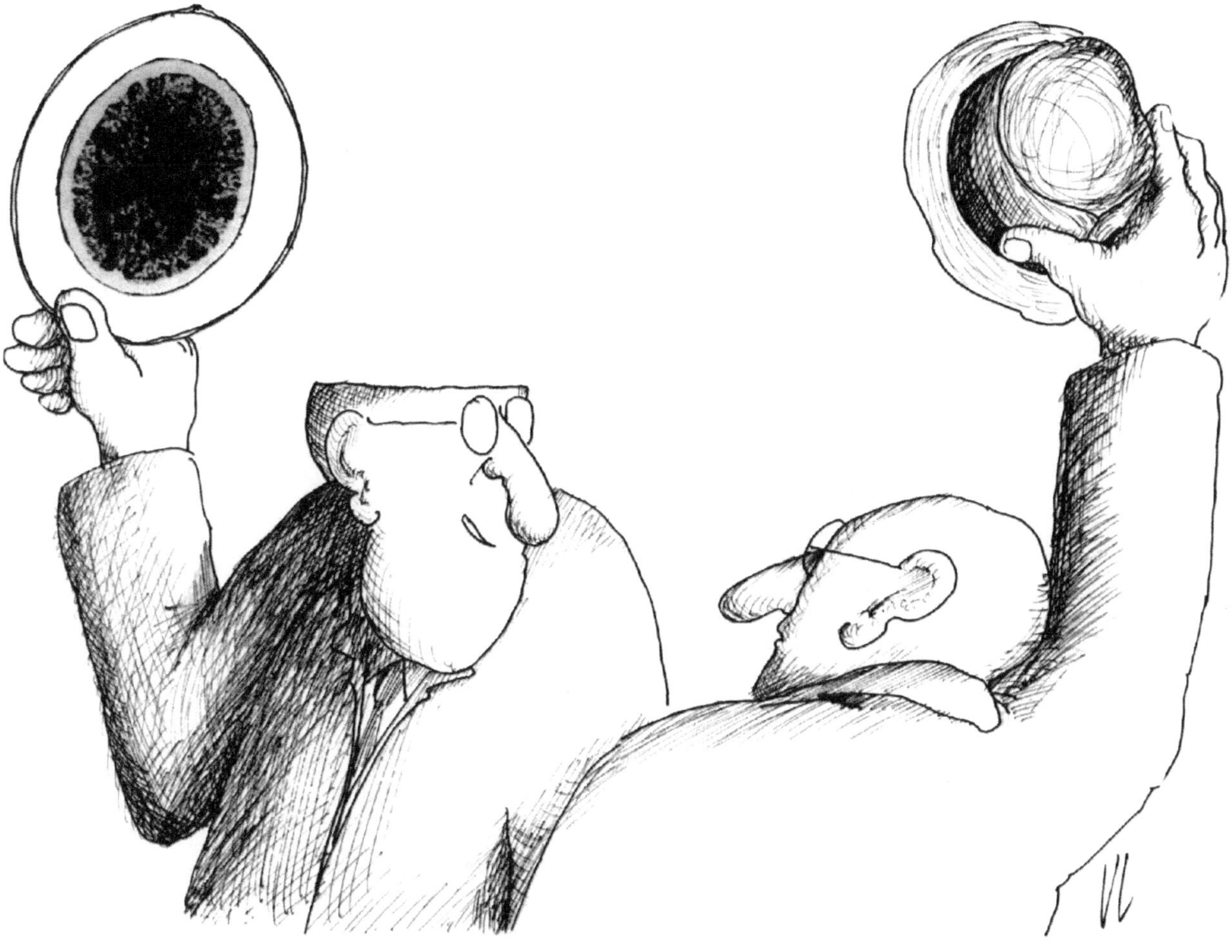

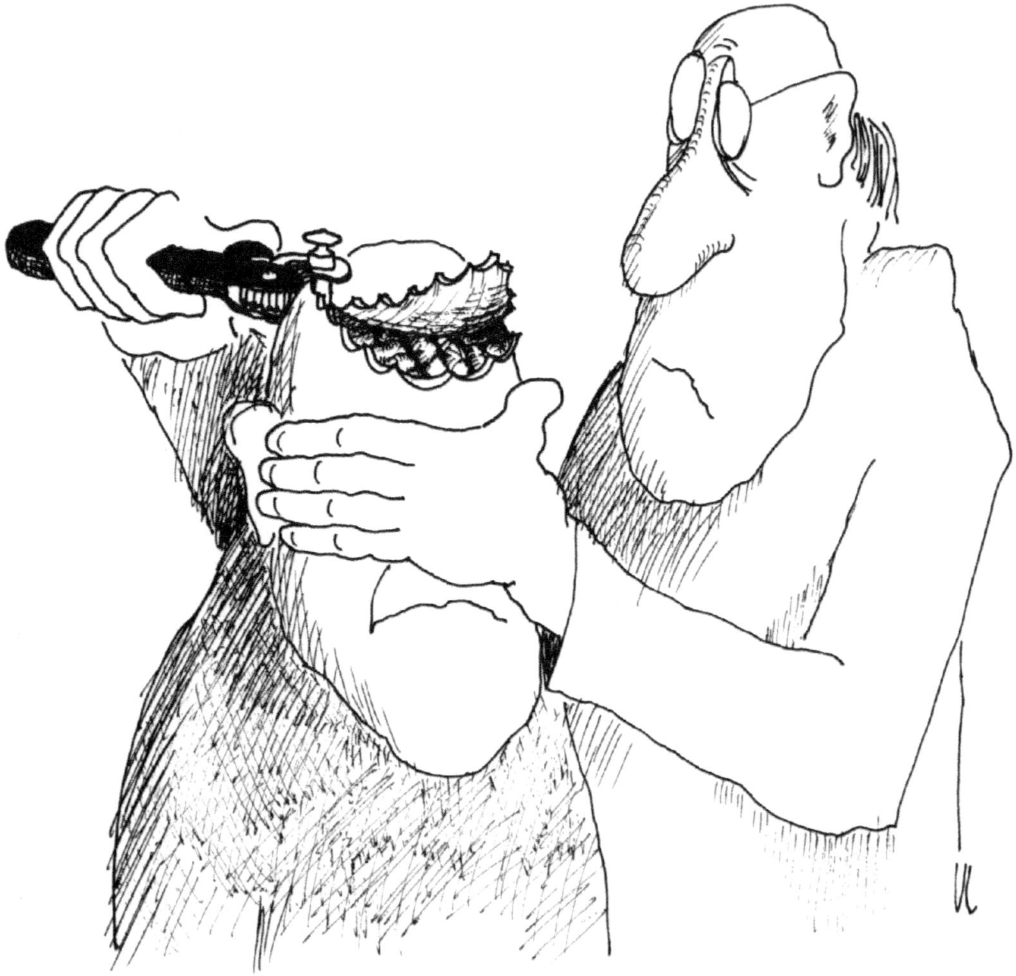

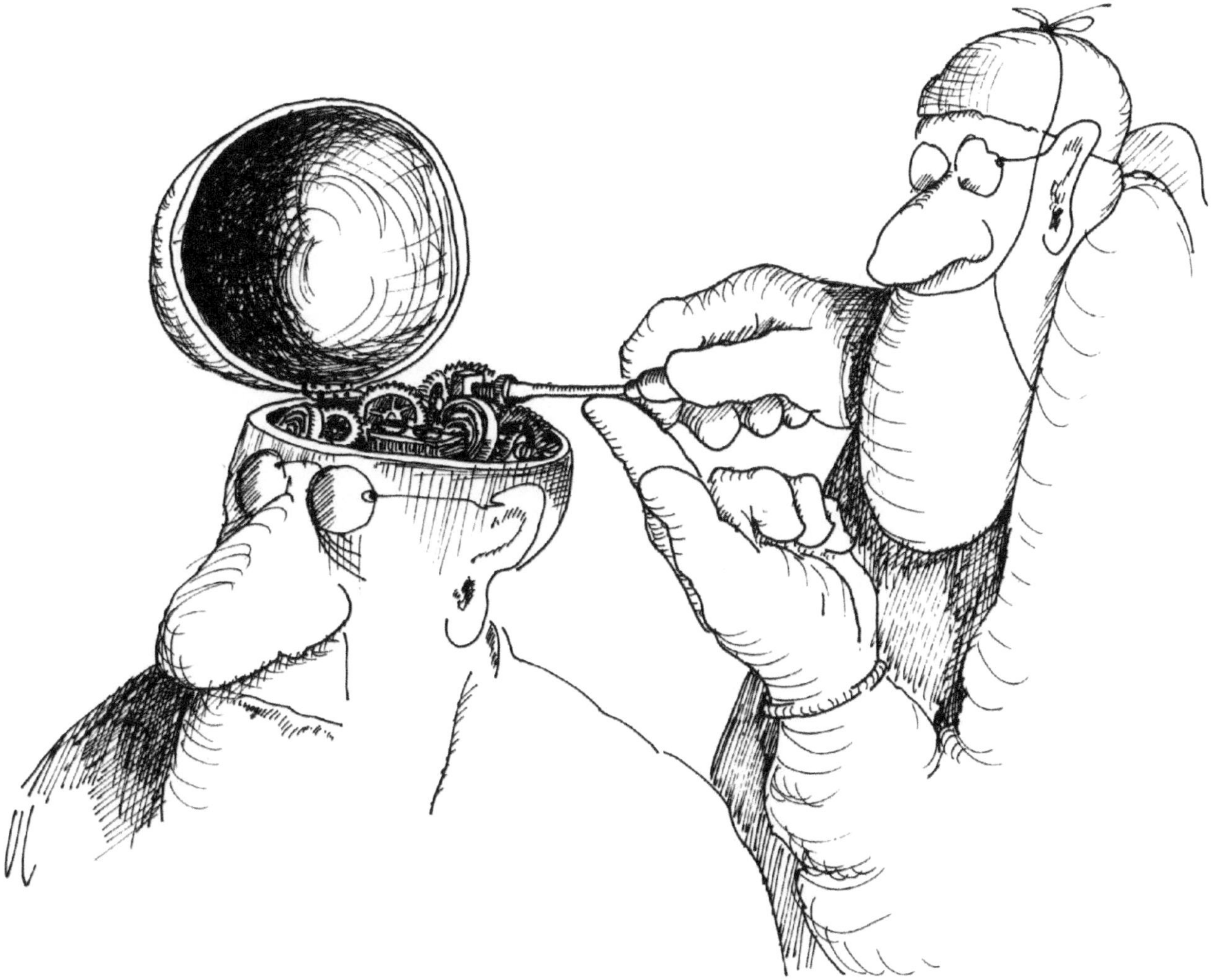

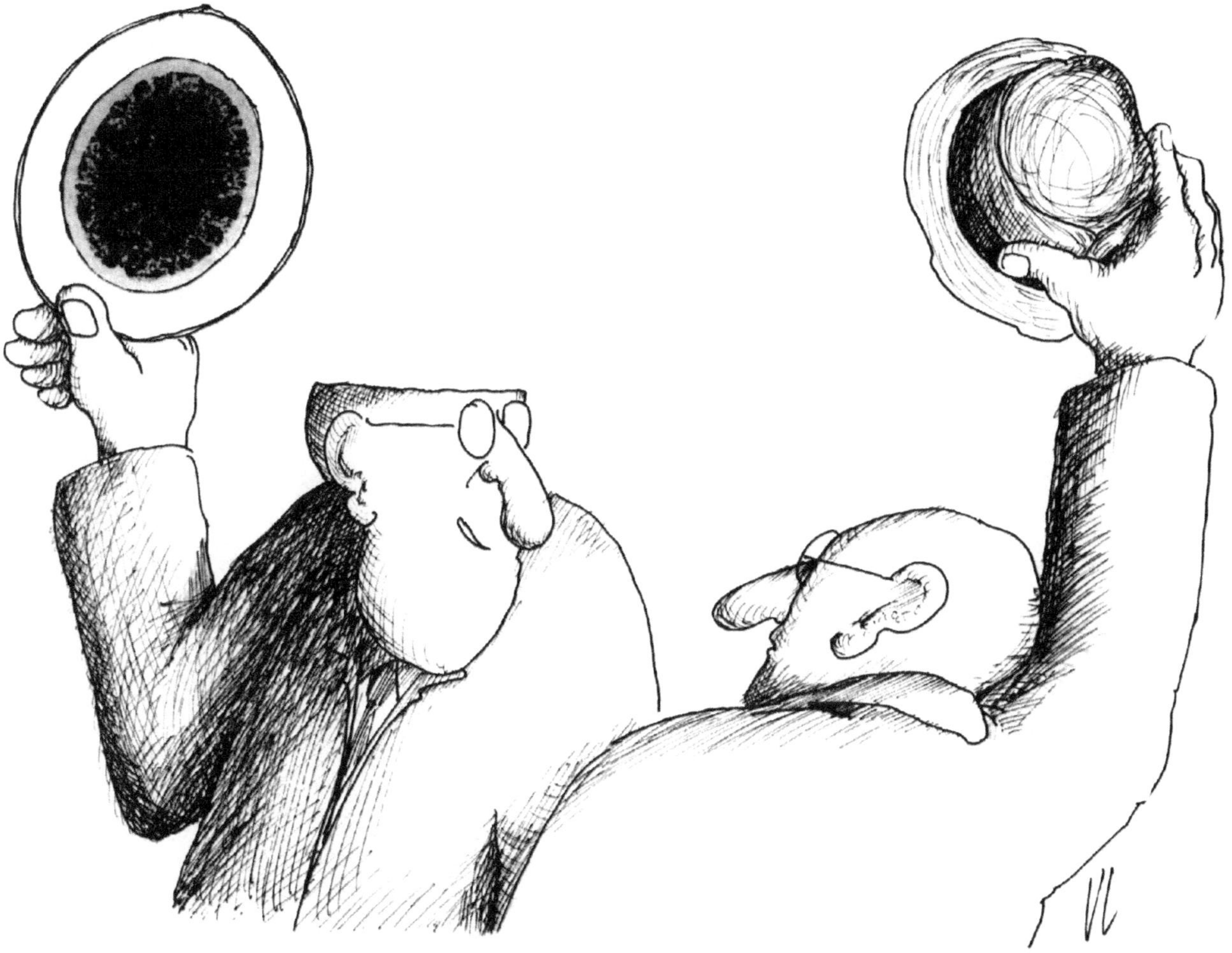

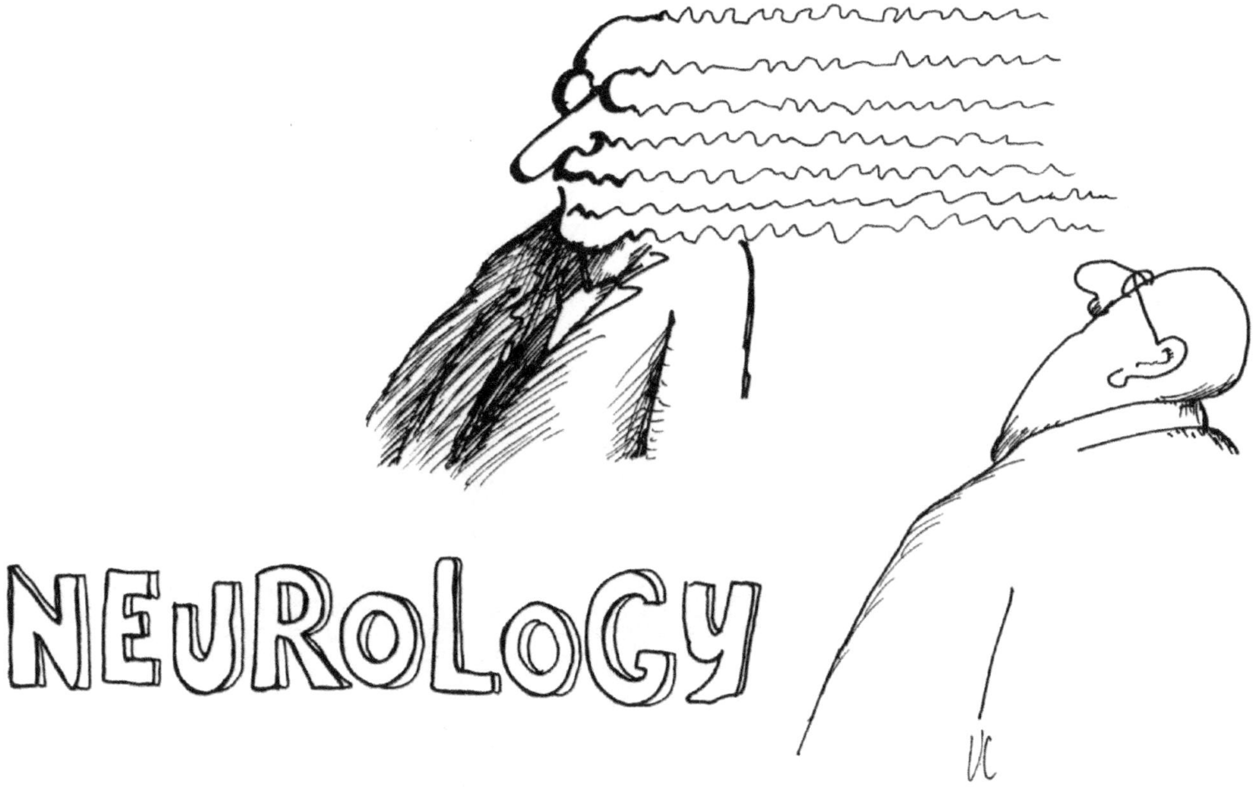
NEUROLOGY

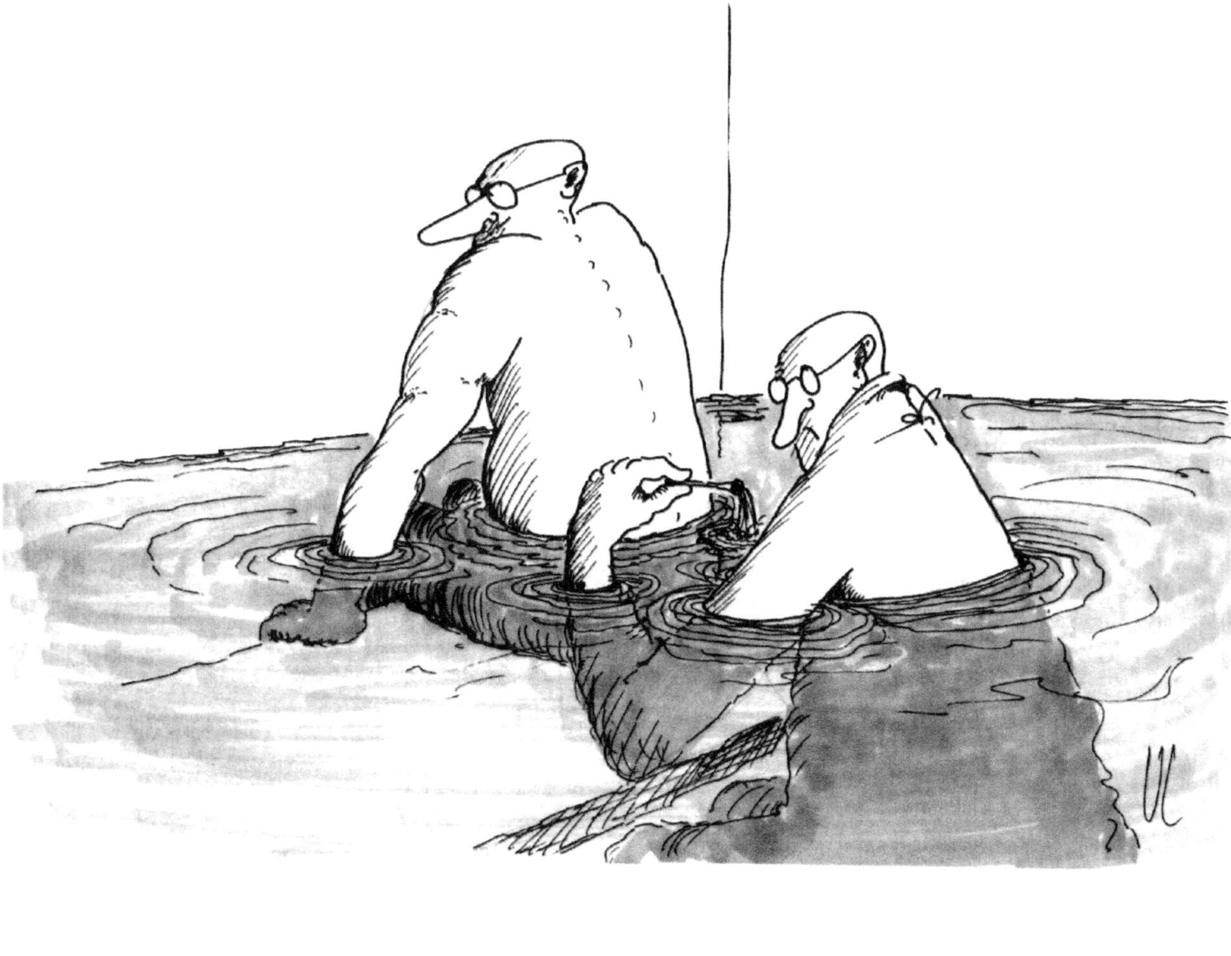

# EMERGENCY MEDICINE

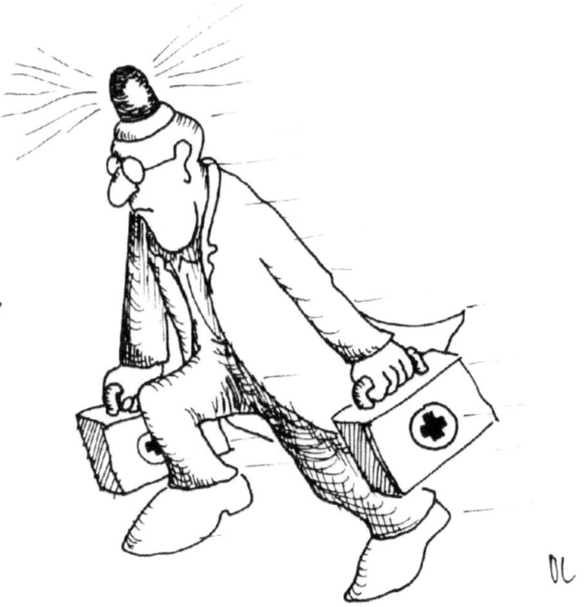

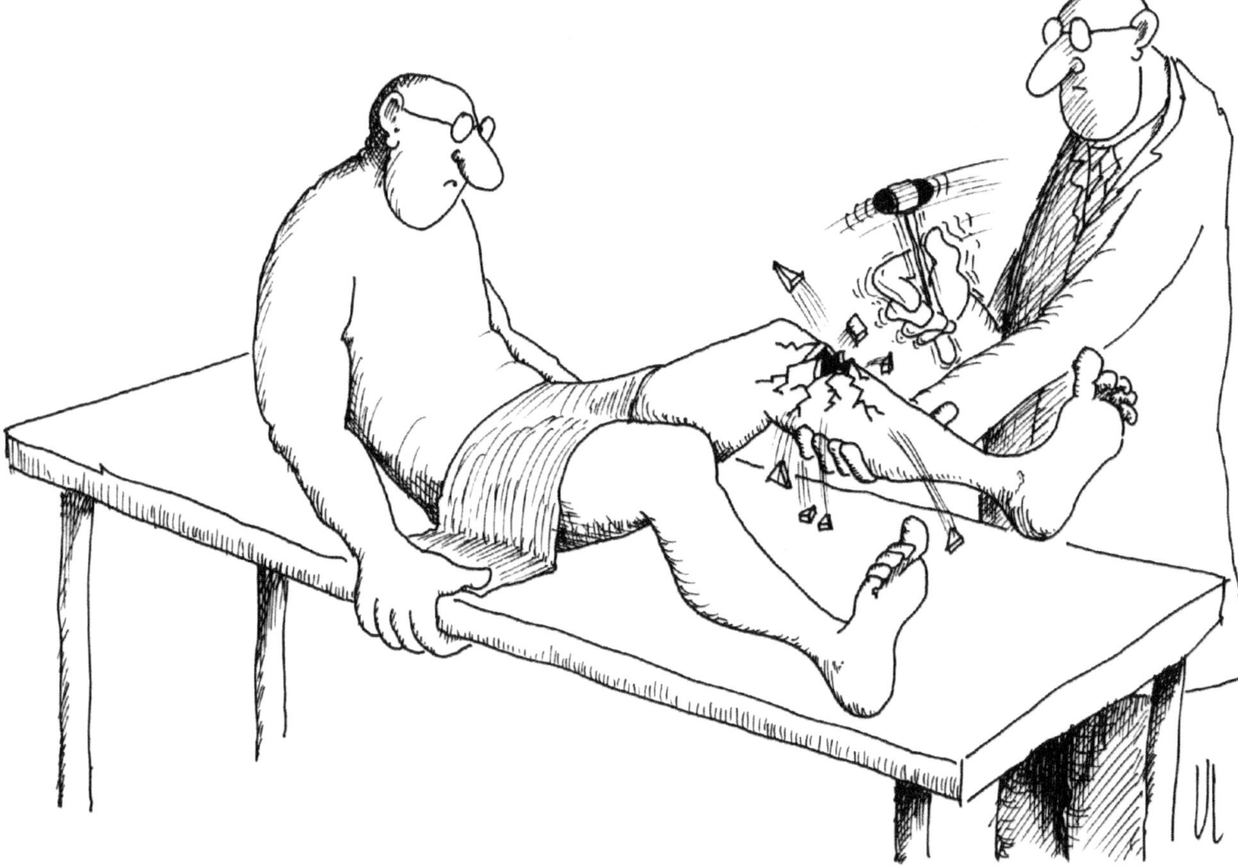

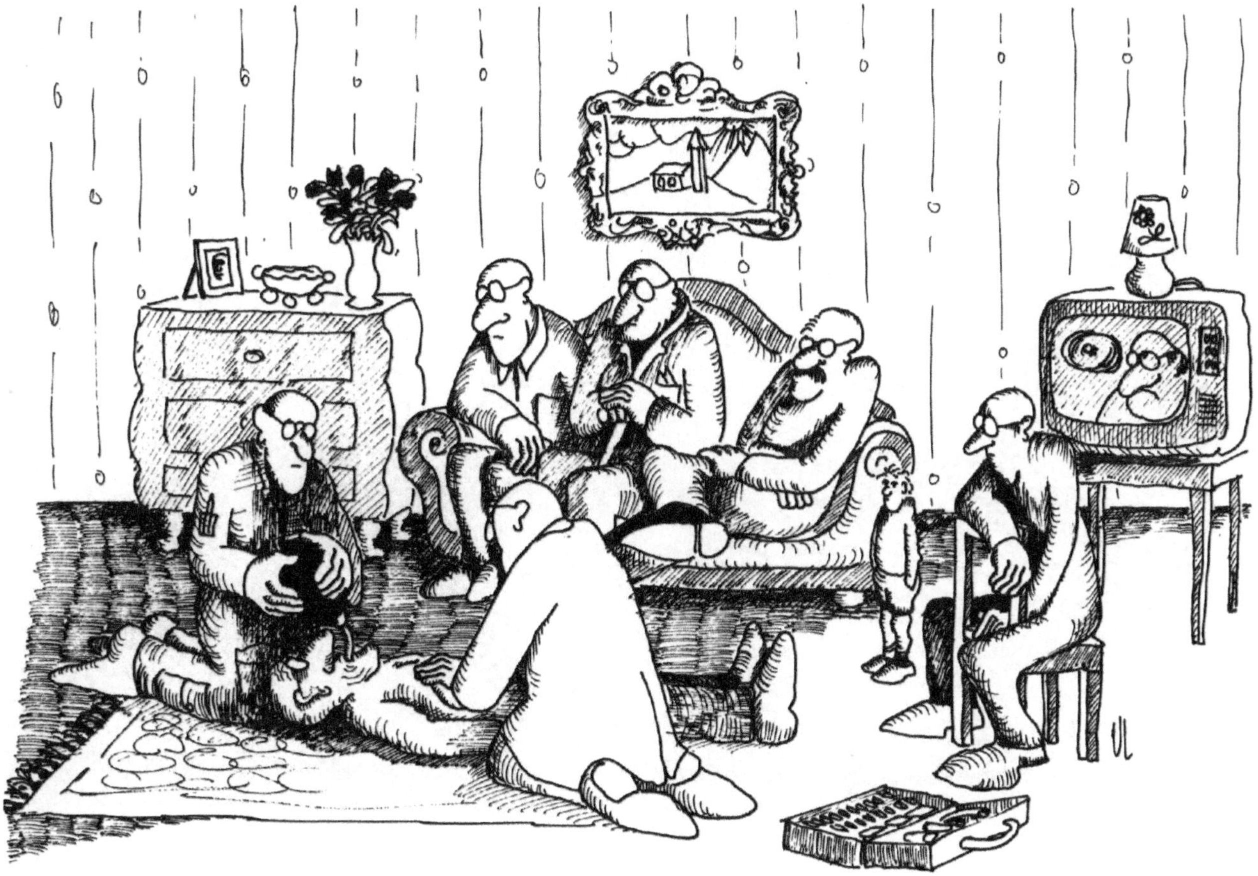

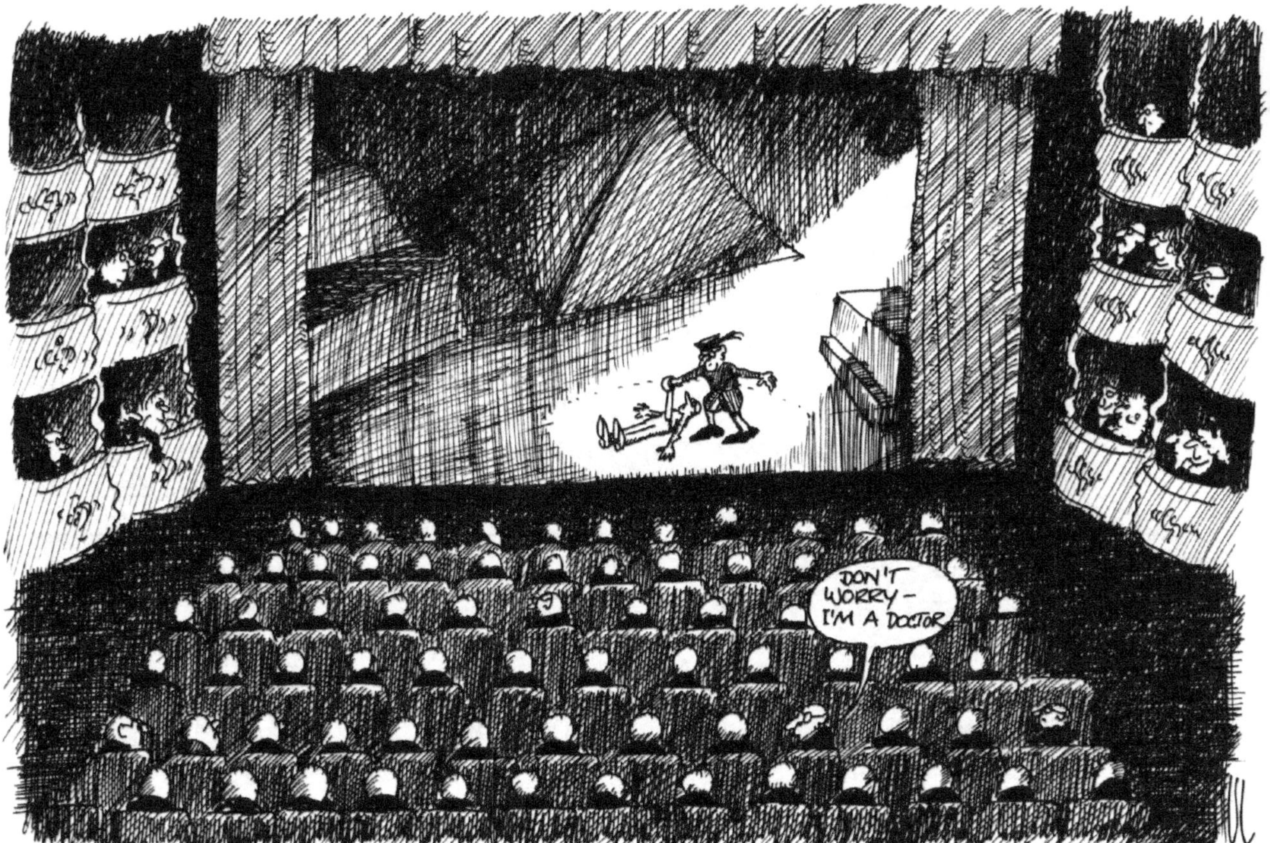
DON'T WORRY - I'M A DOCTOR

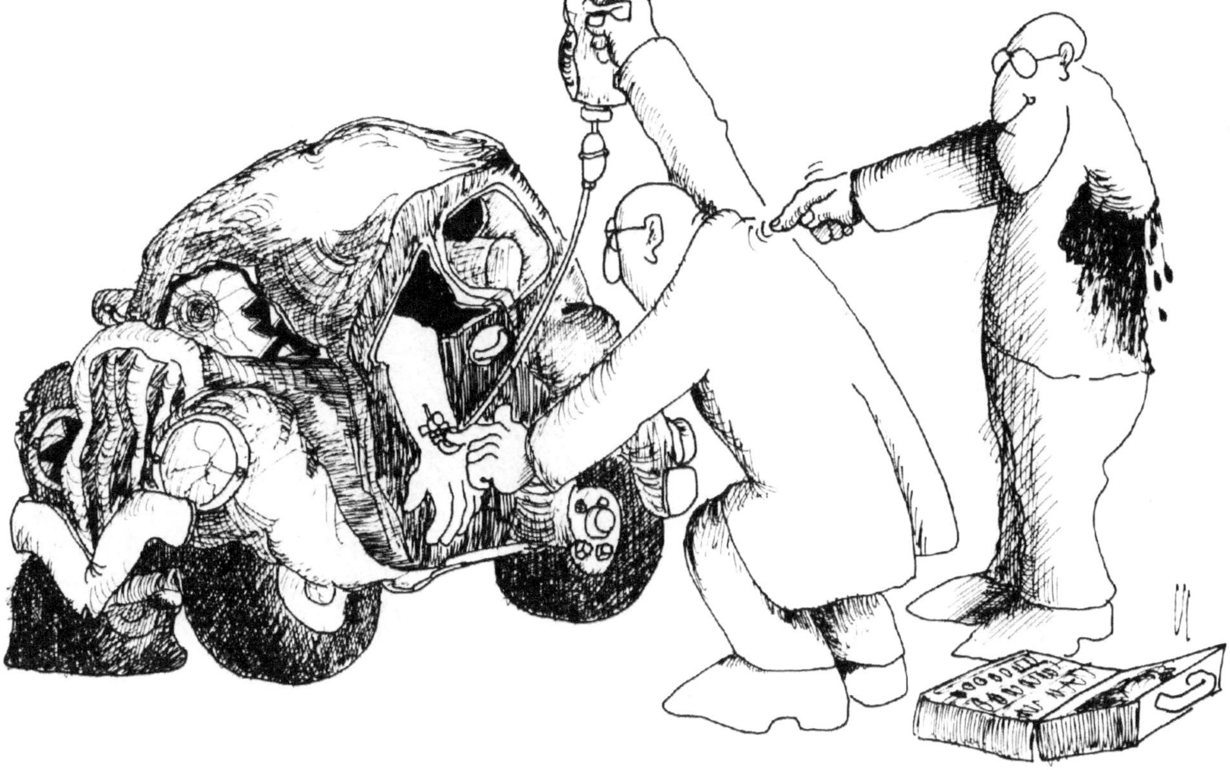

# OPHTHAL-MOLOGY

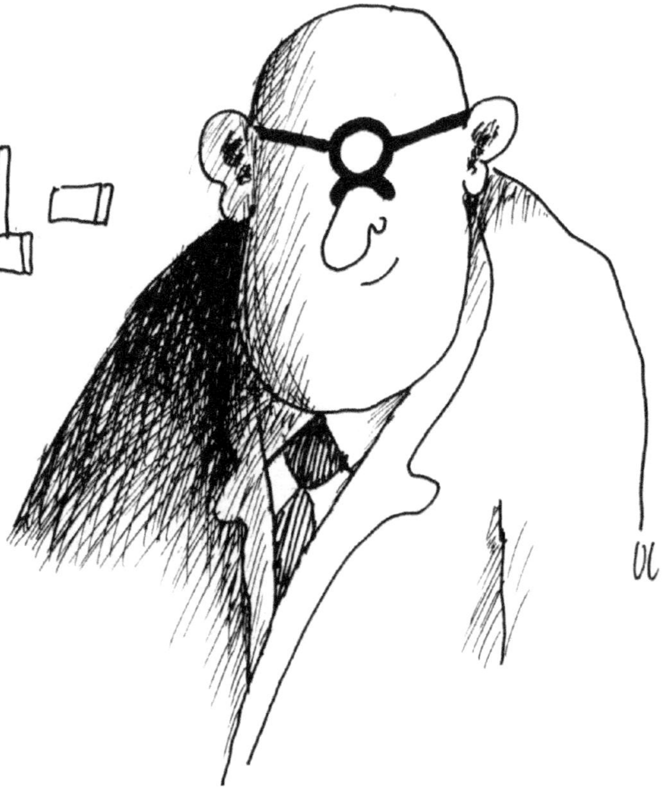

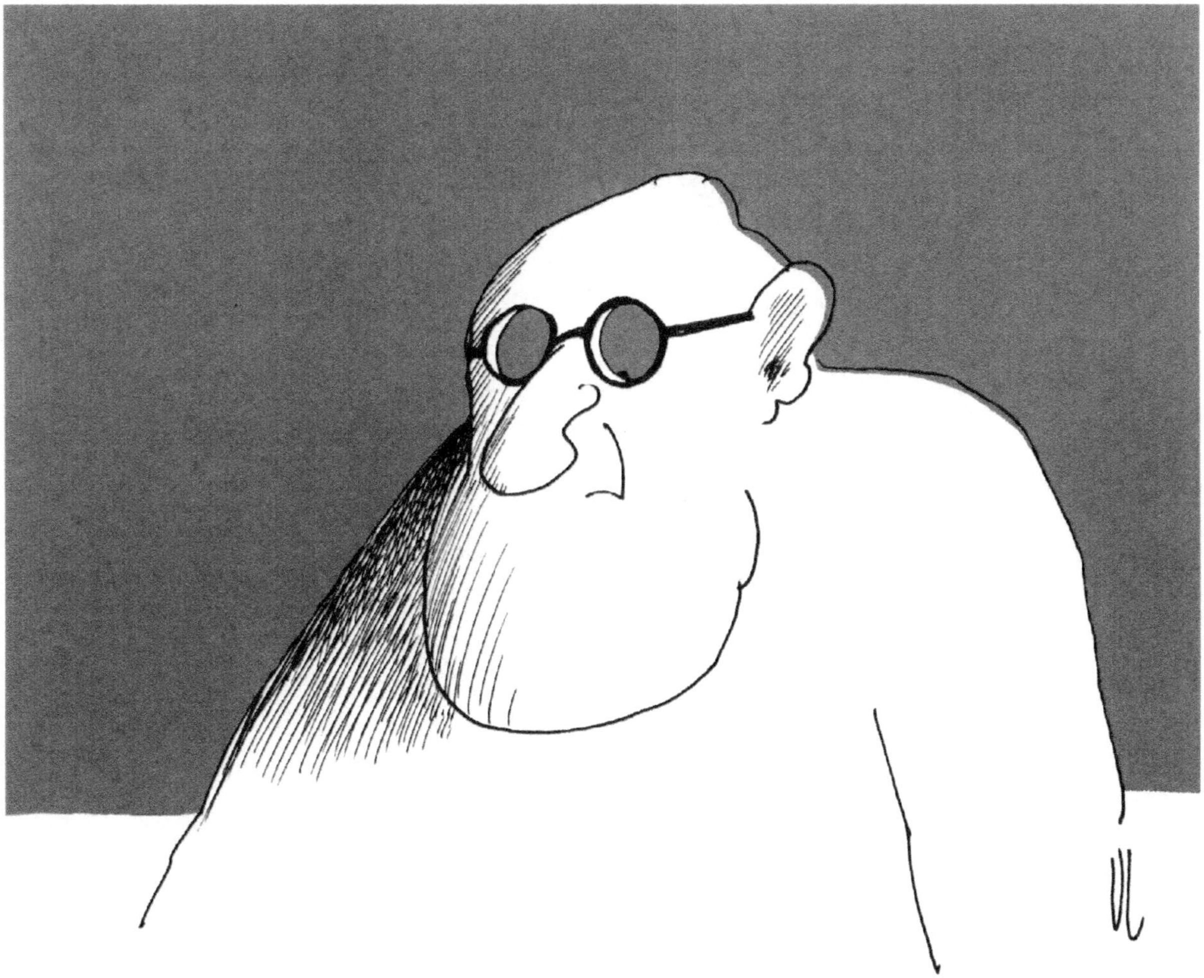

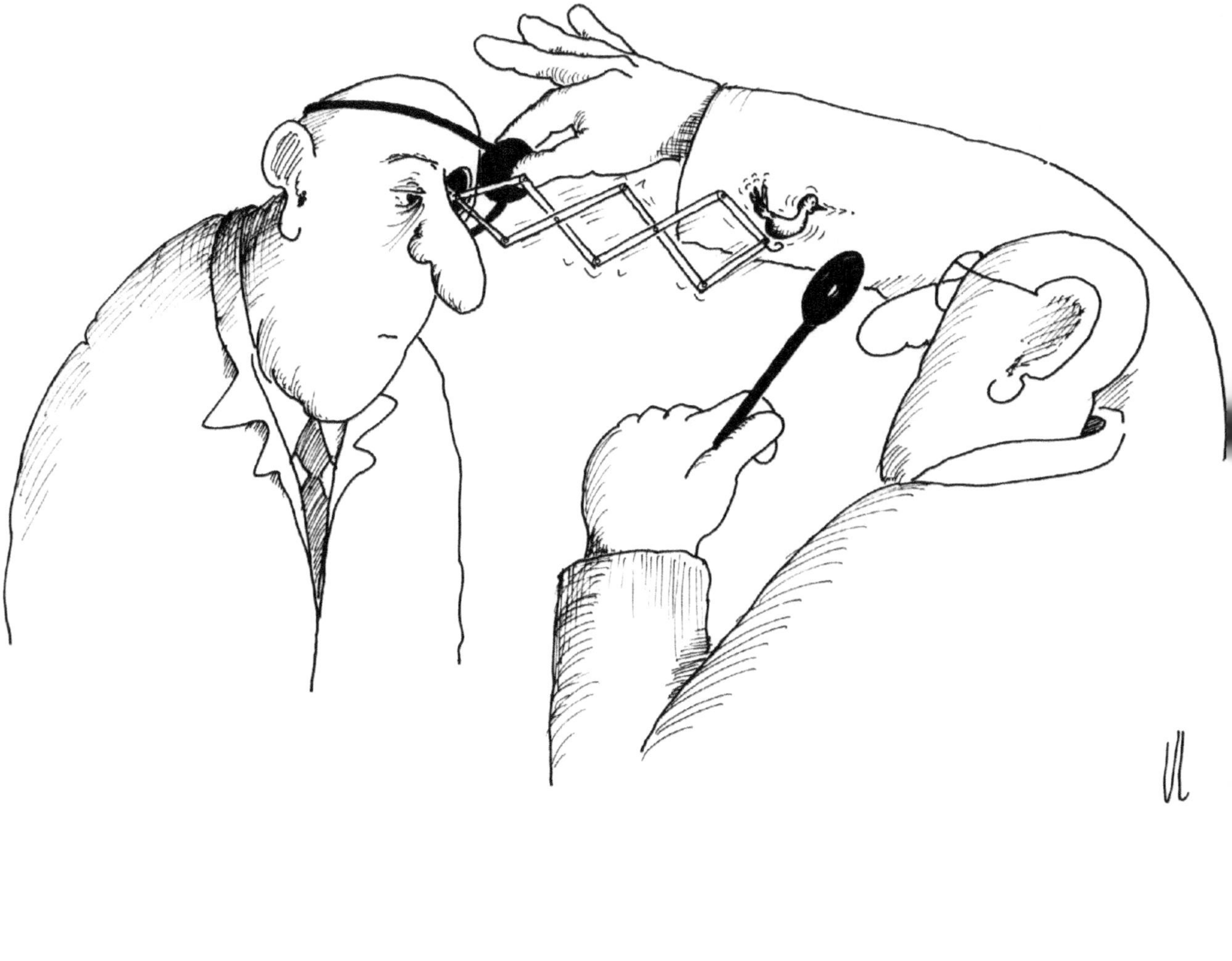

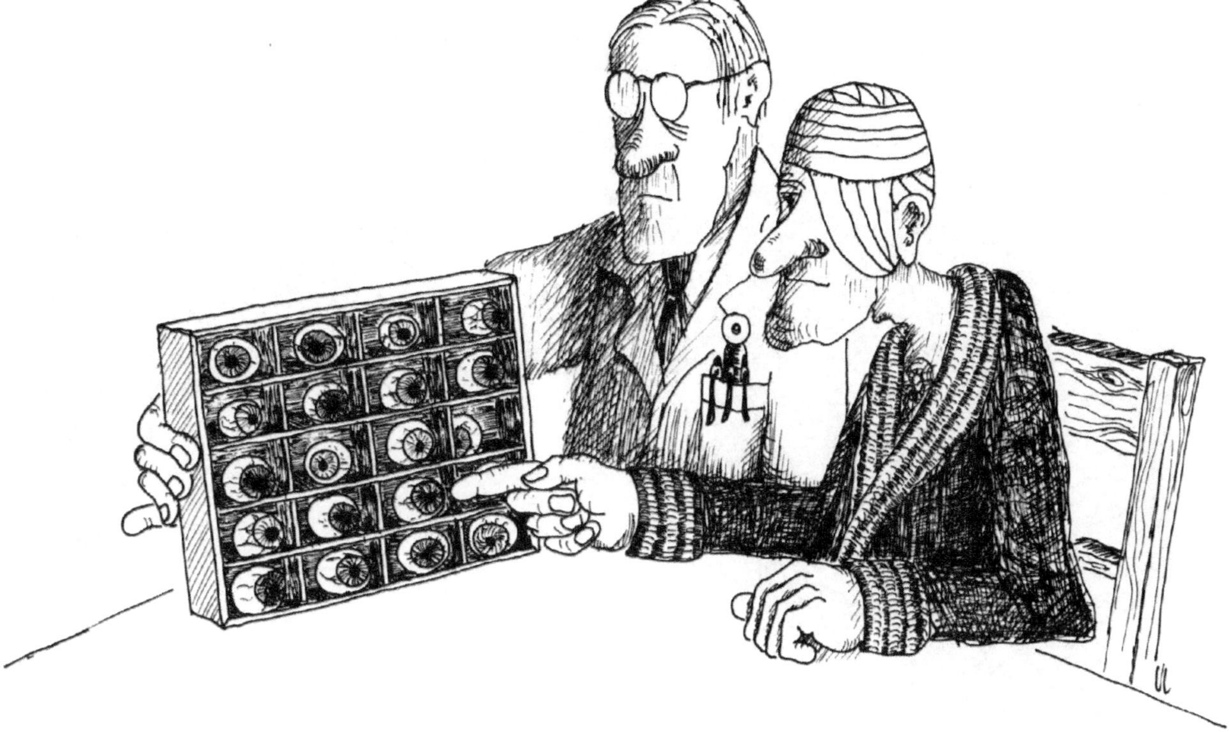

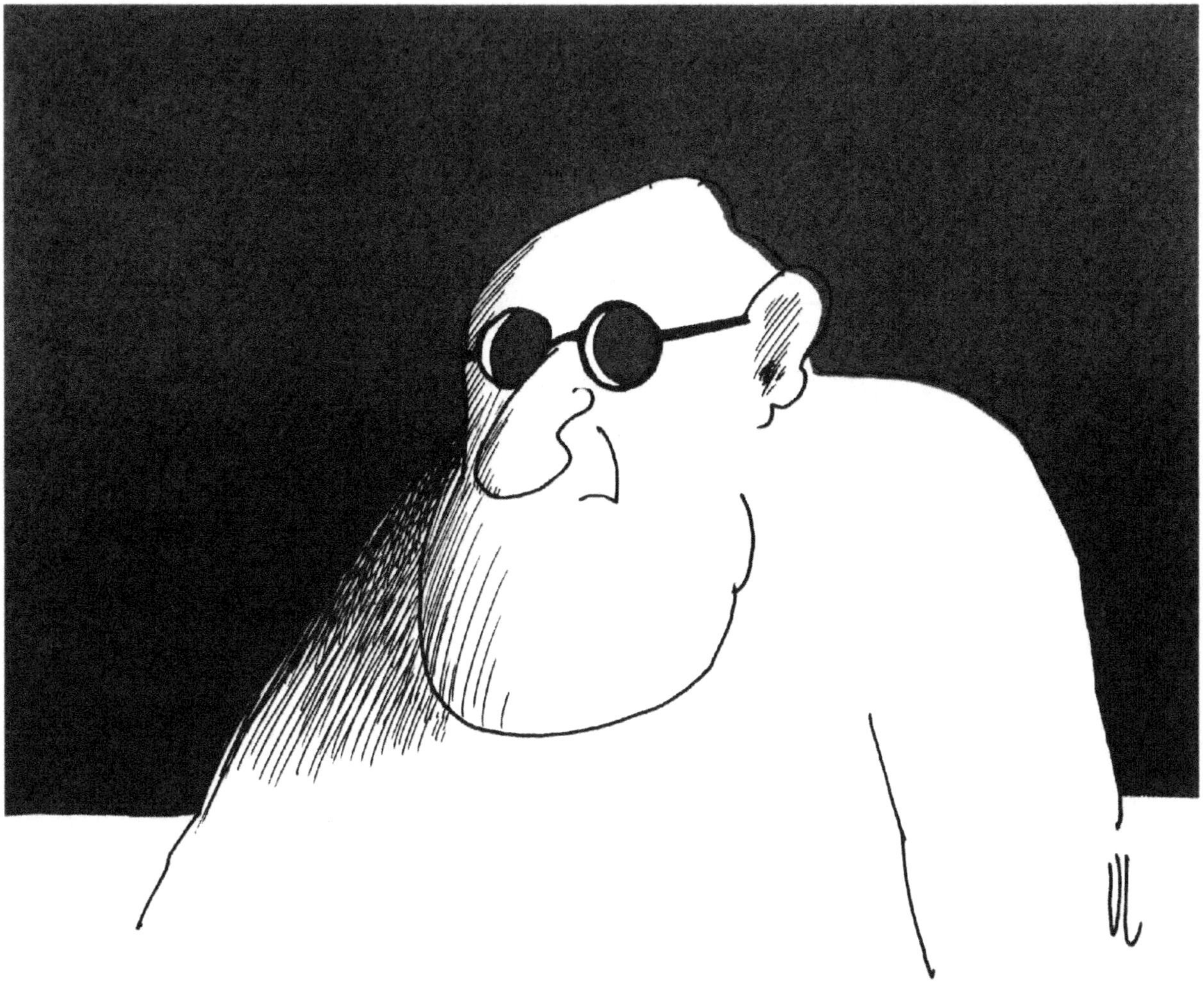

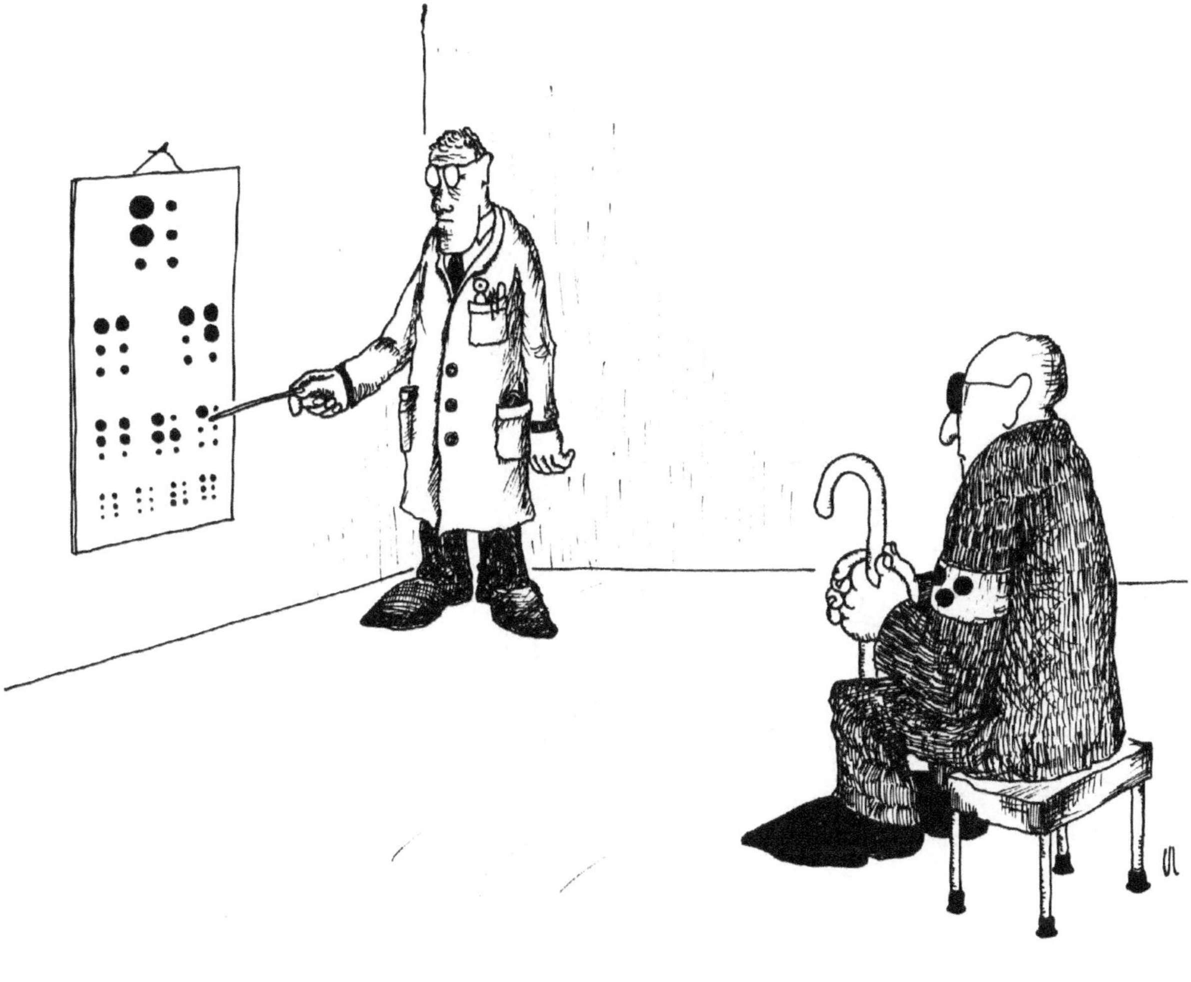

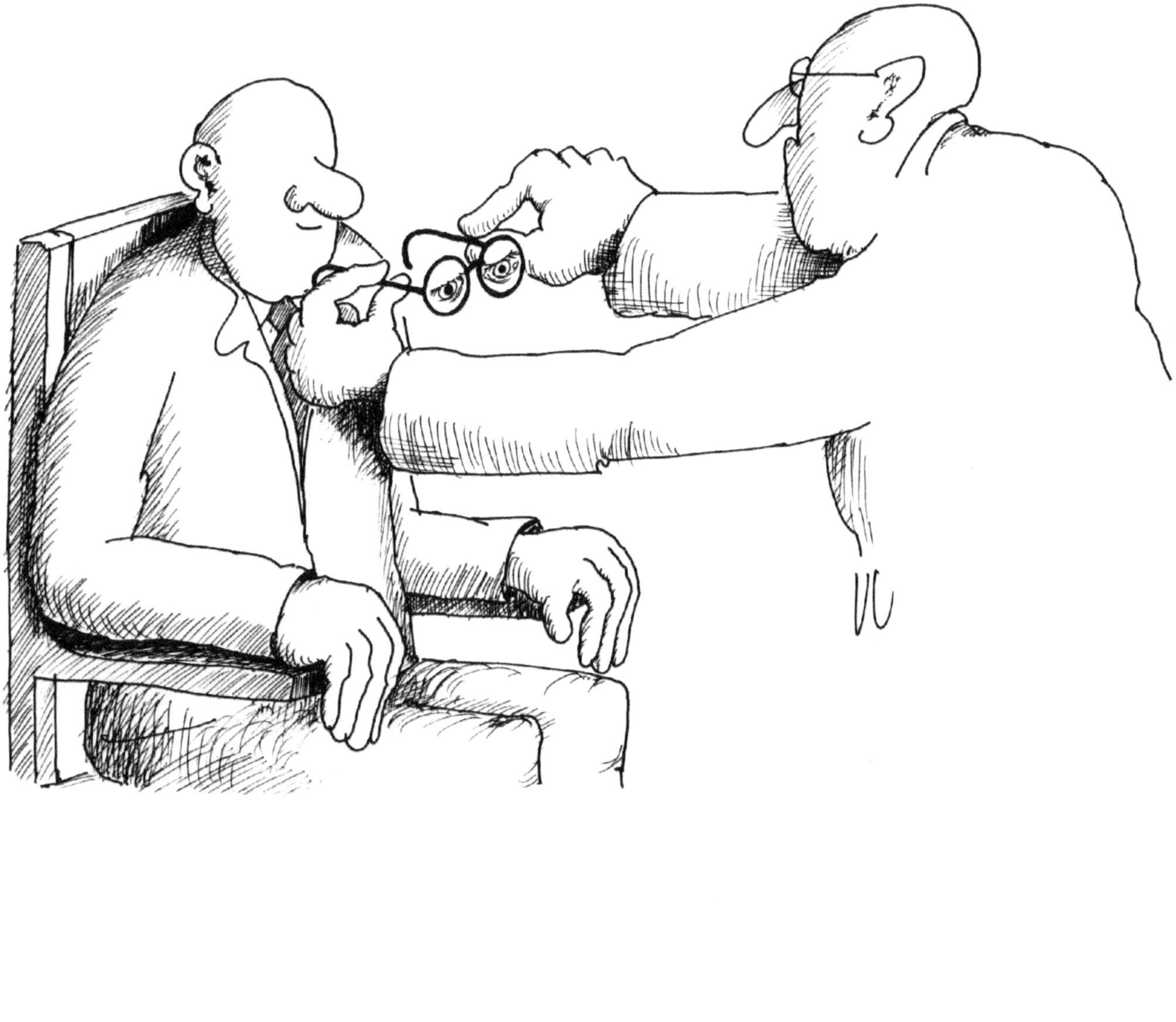

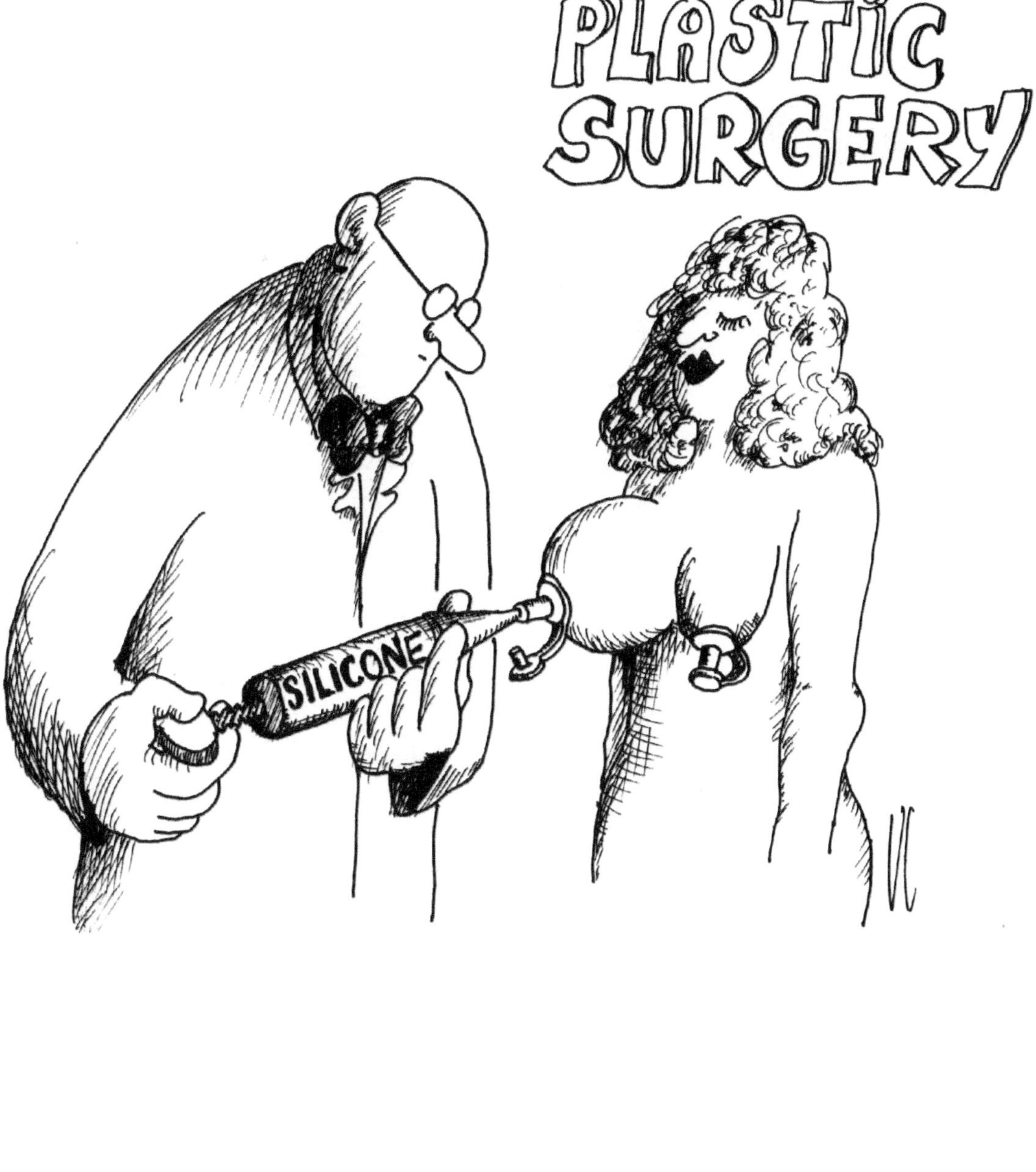
PLASTIC SURGERY
SILICONE

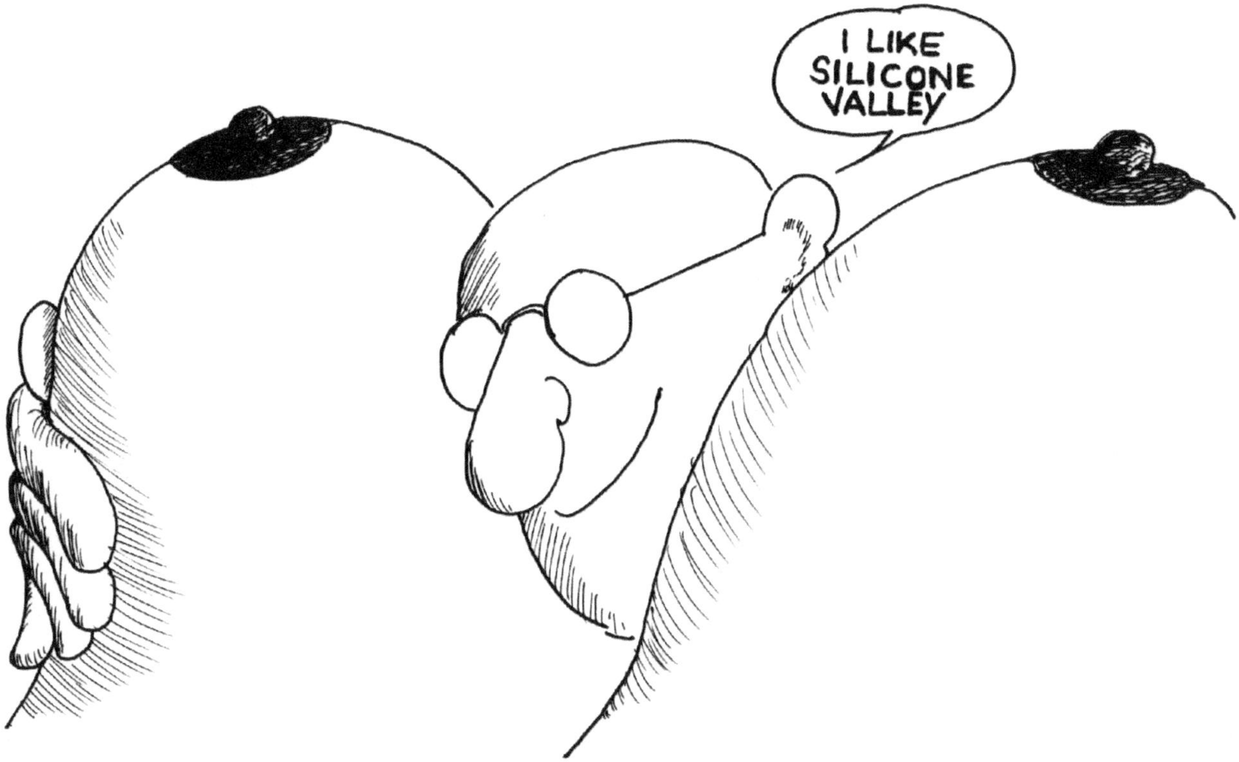
I LIKE SILICONE VALLEY

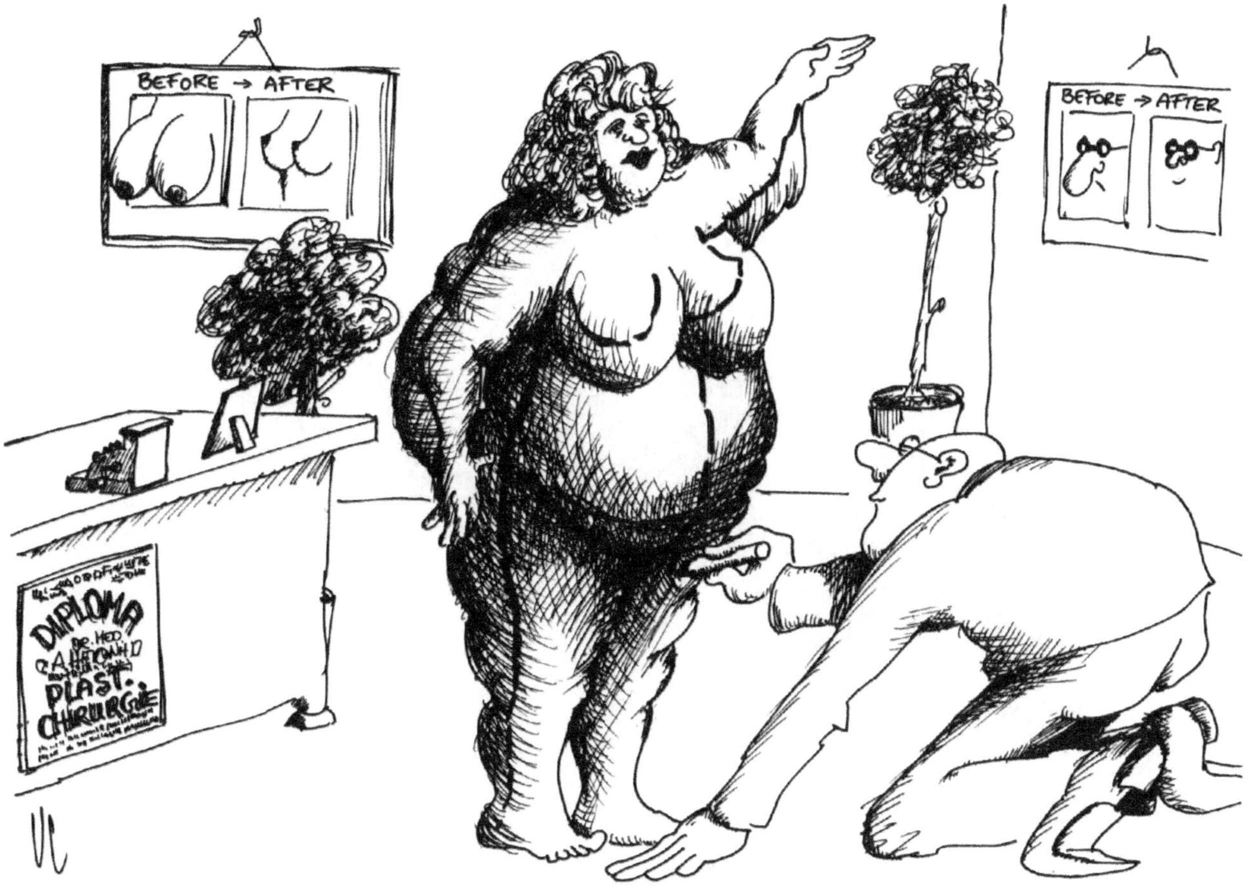
BEFORE → AFTER
BEFORE → AFTER
DIPLOMA
DR. MED
PLAST.
CHIRURGIE

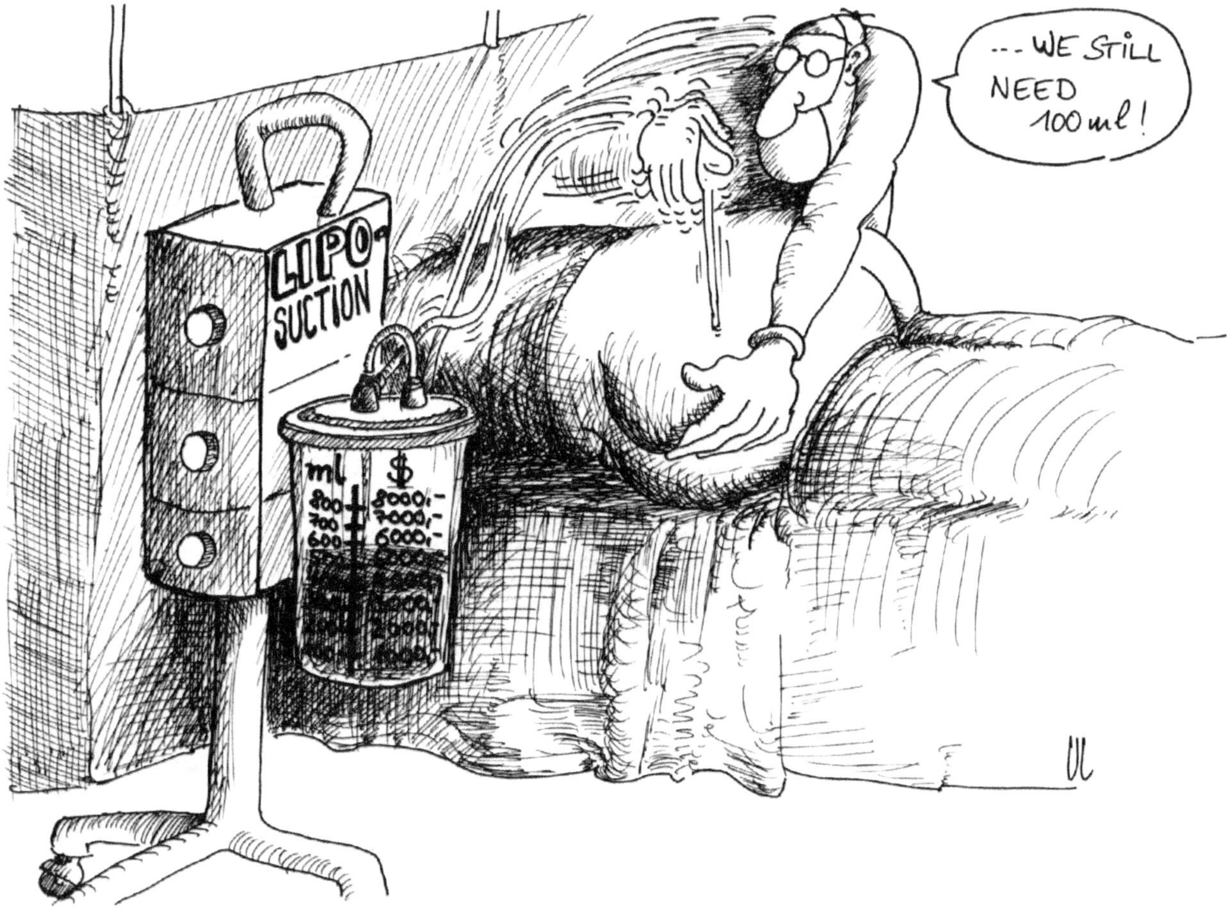
LIPO-SUCTION
ml
$
800
700
600
8000,-
7000,-
6000,-
--- WE STILL NEED 100 ml!

# PROCTOLOGY

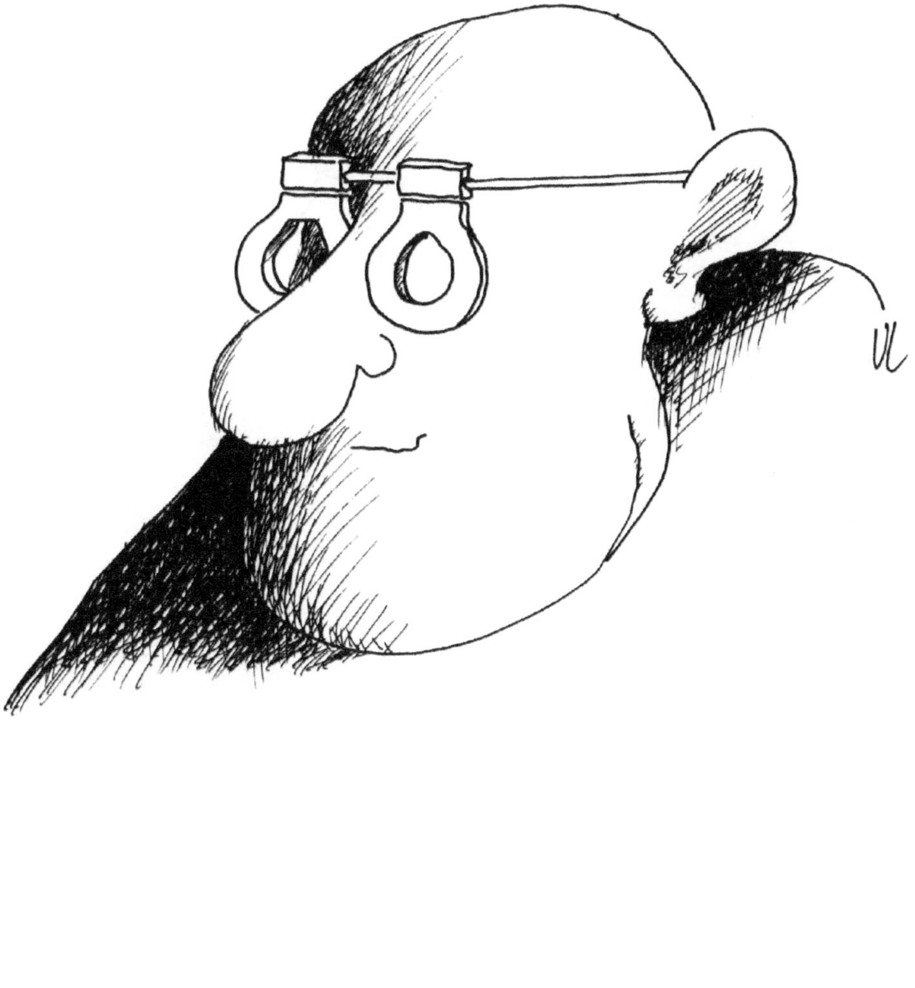

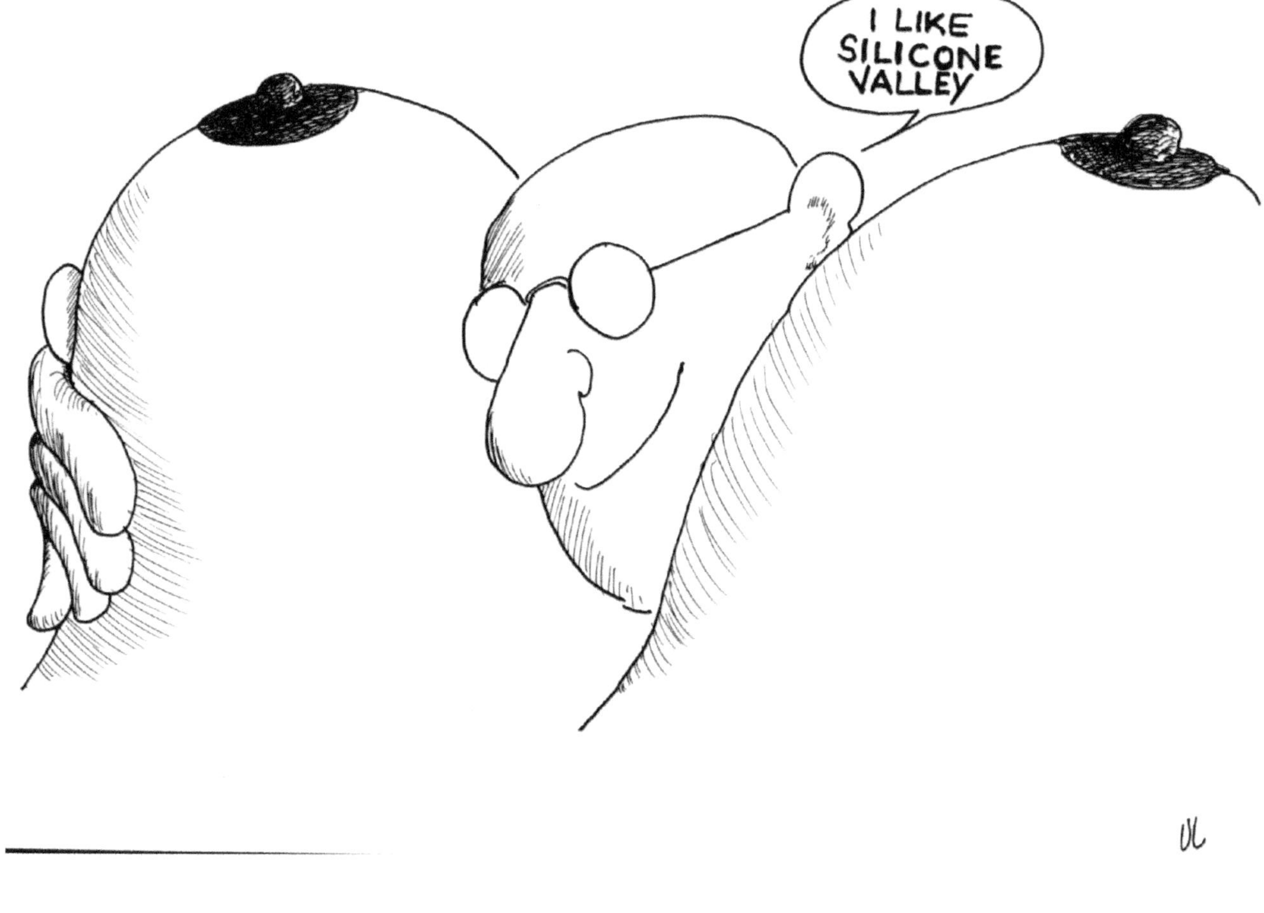
I LIKE SILICONE VALLEY

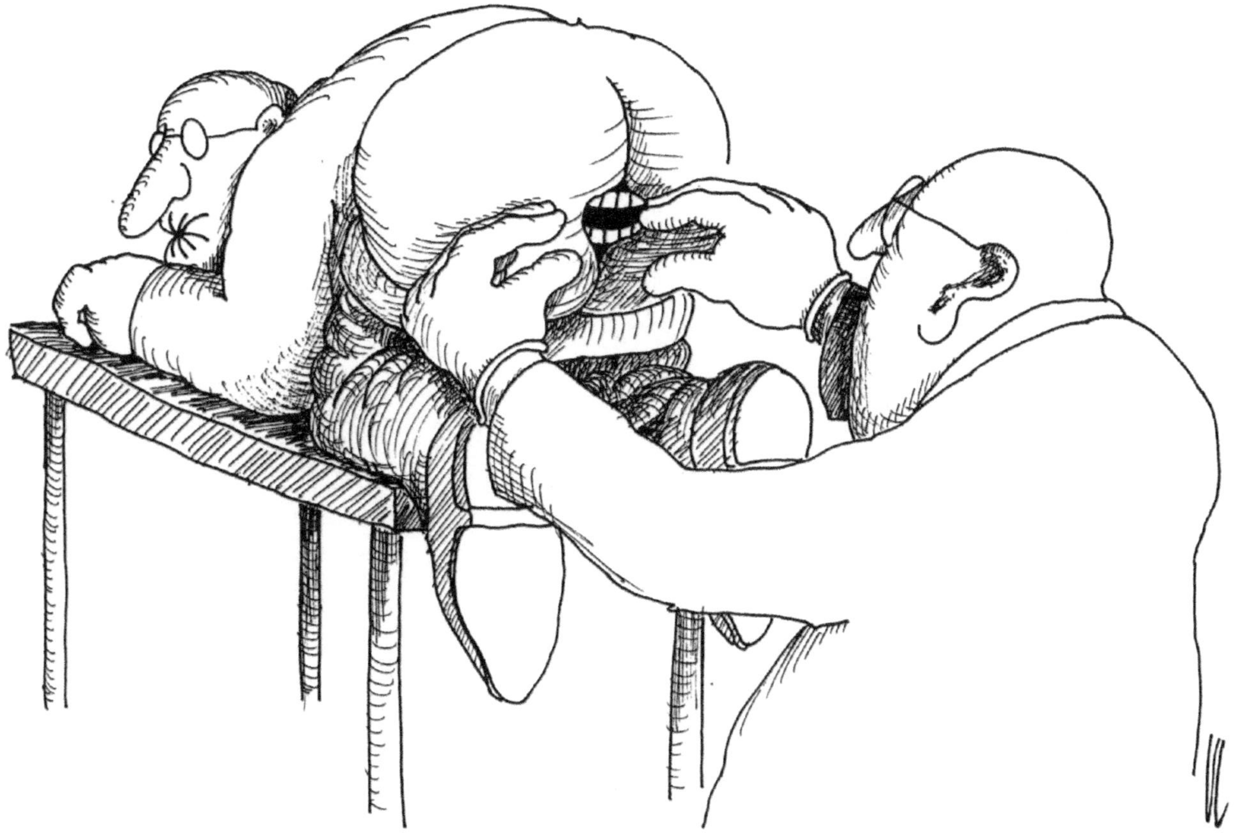

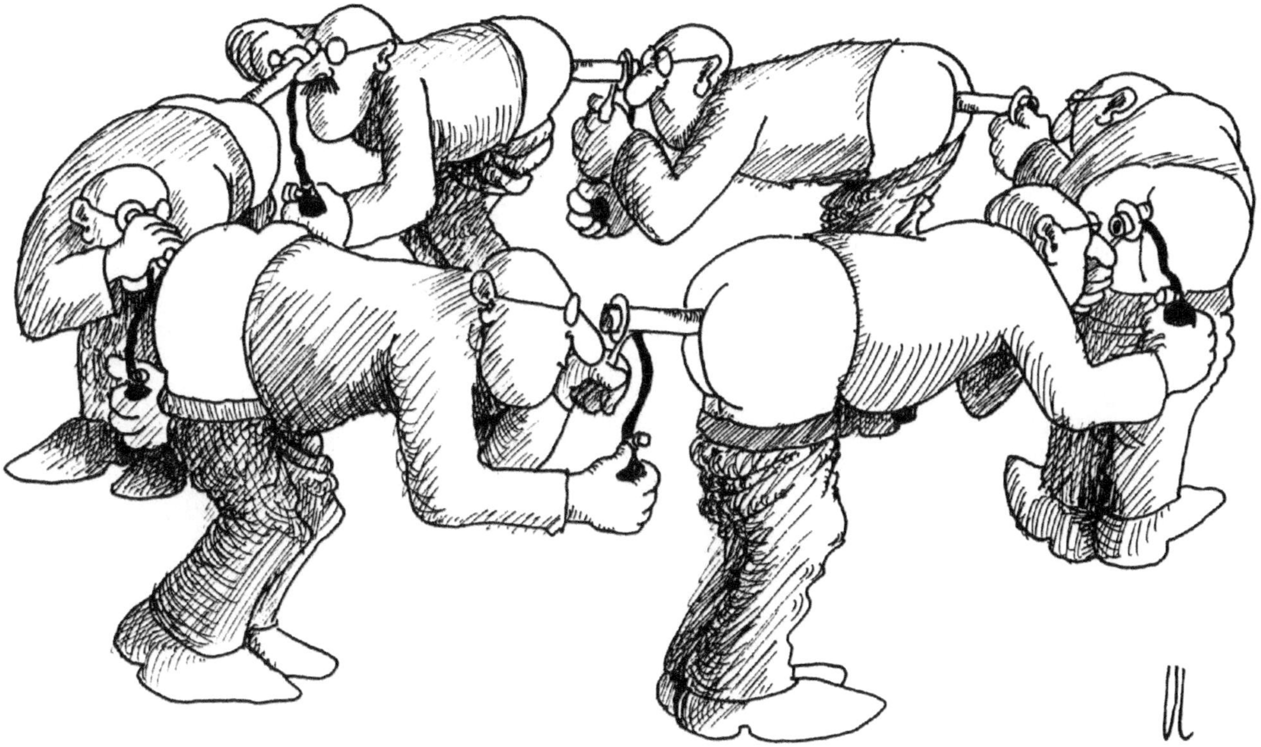

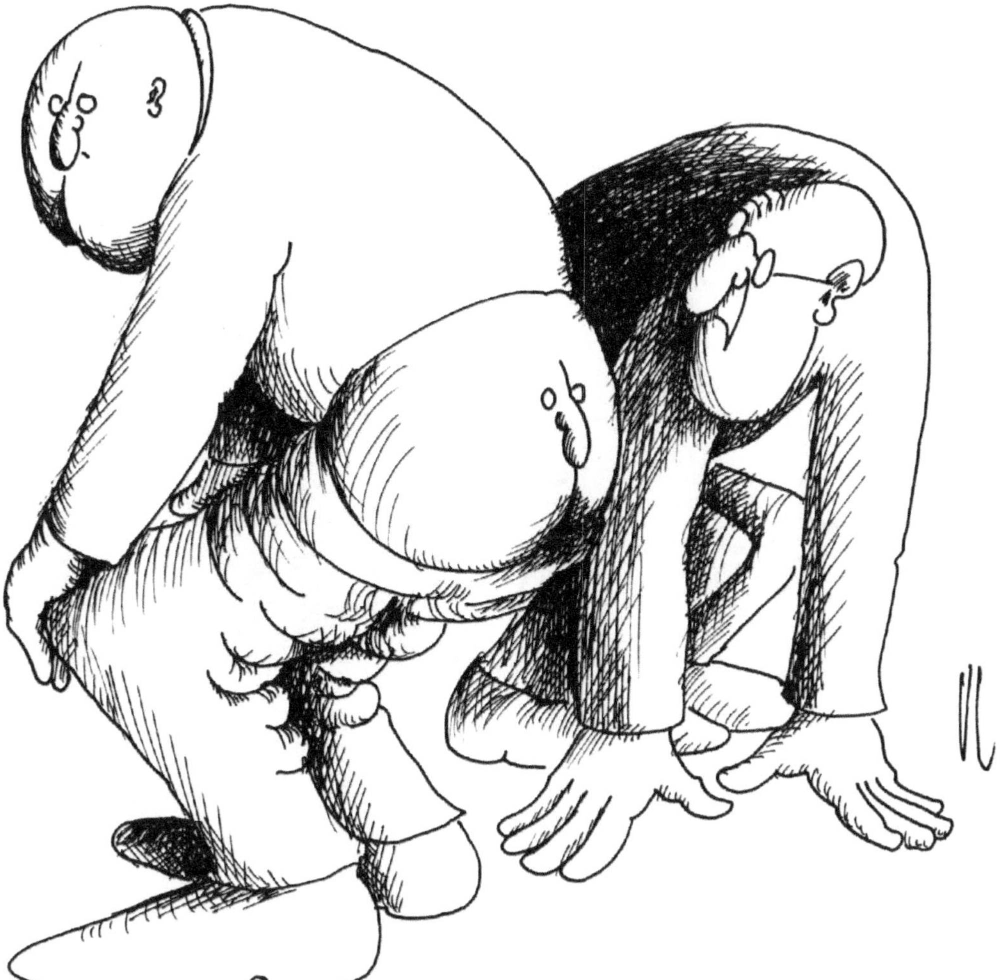

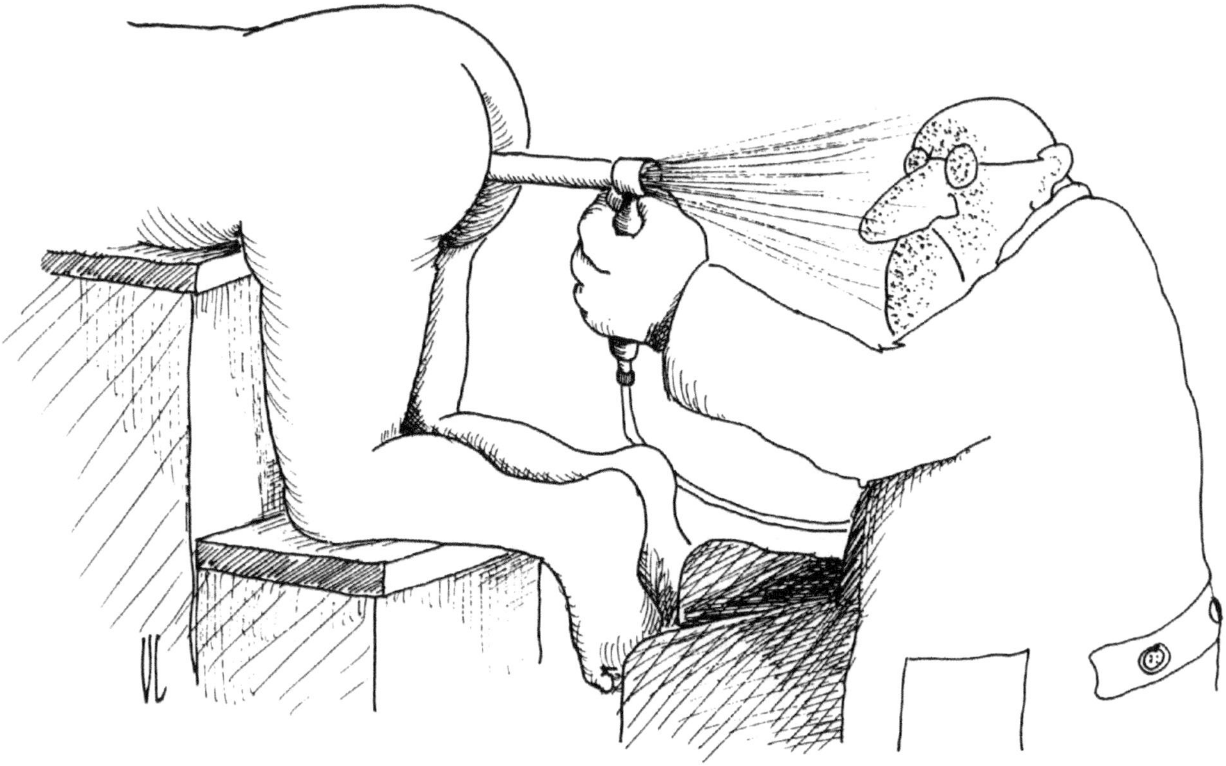
VL

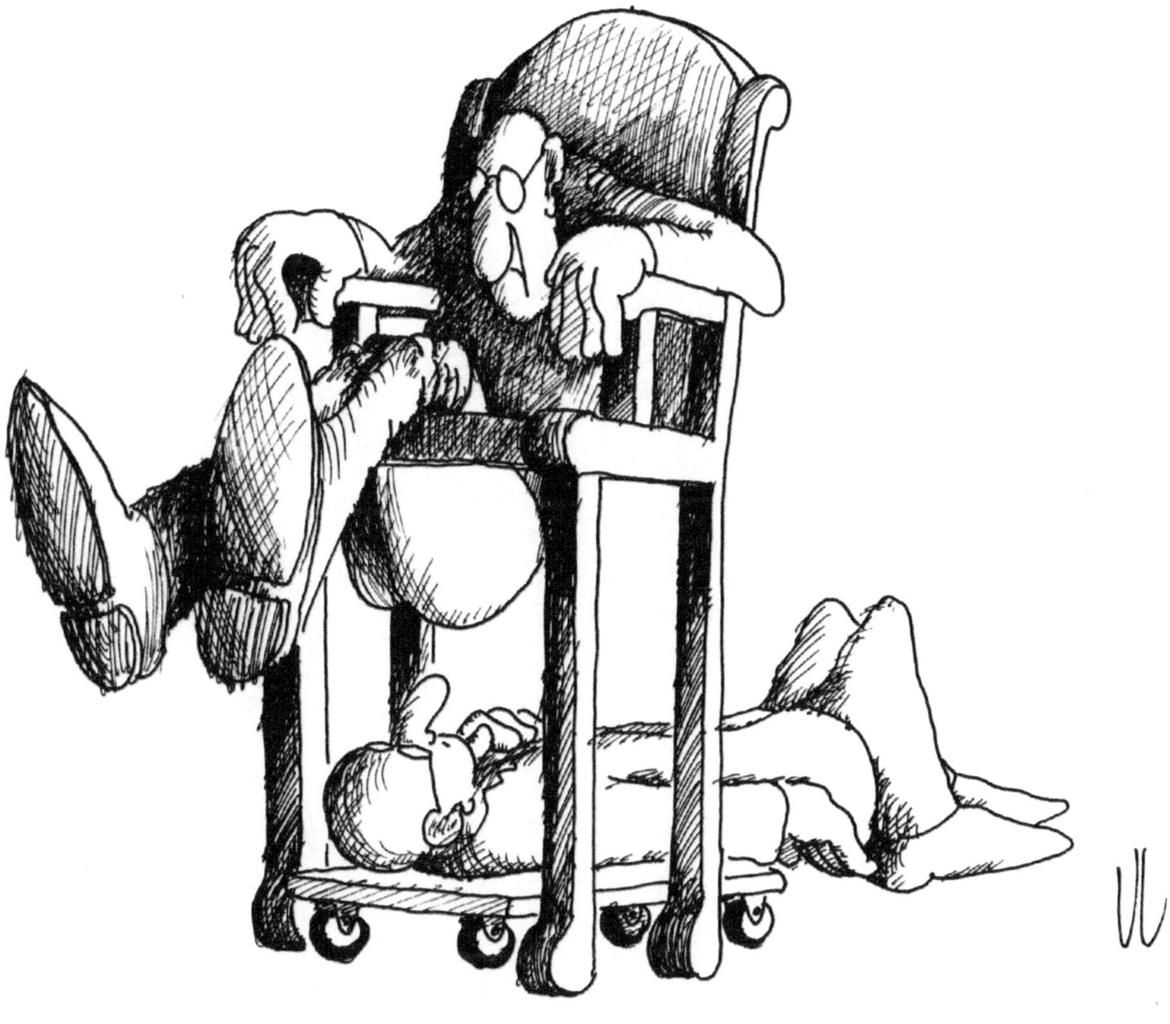

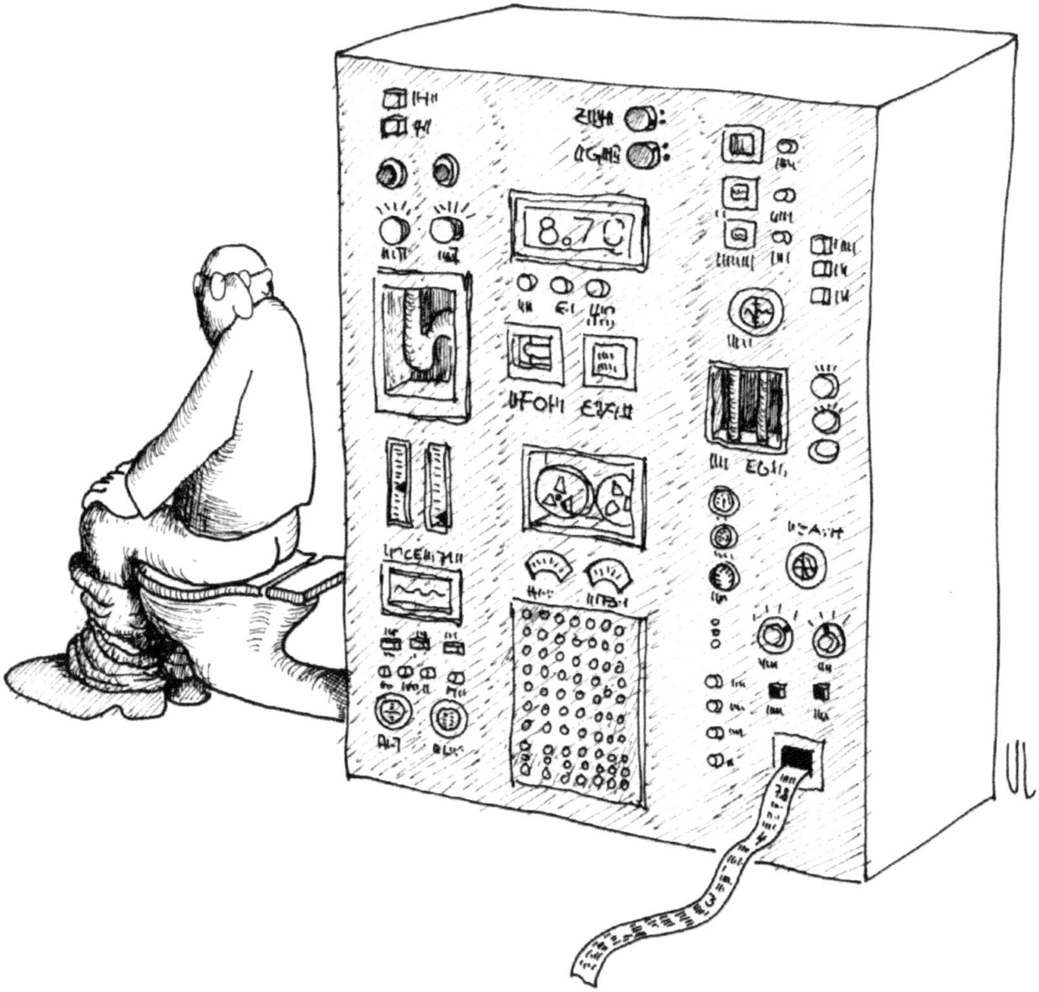

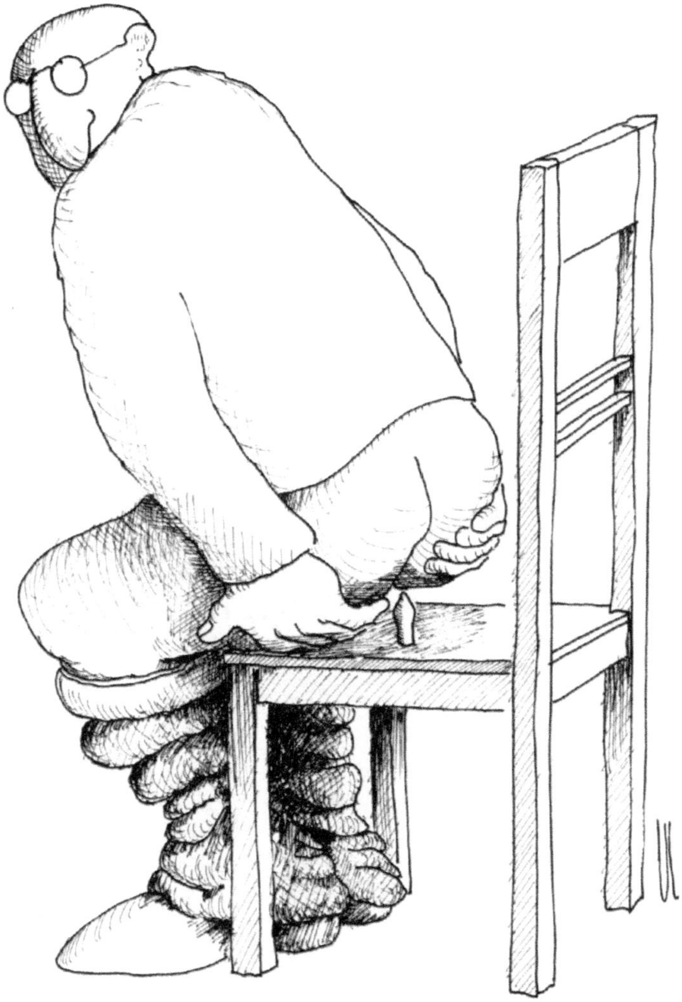

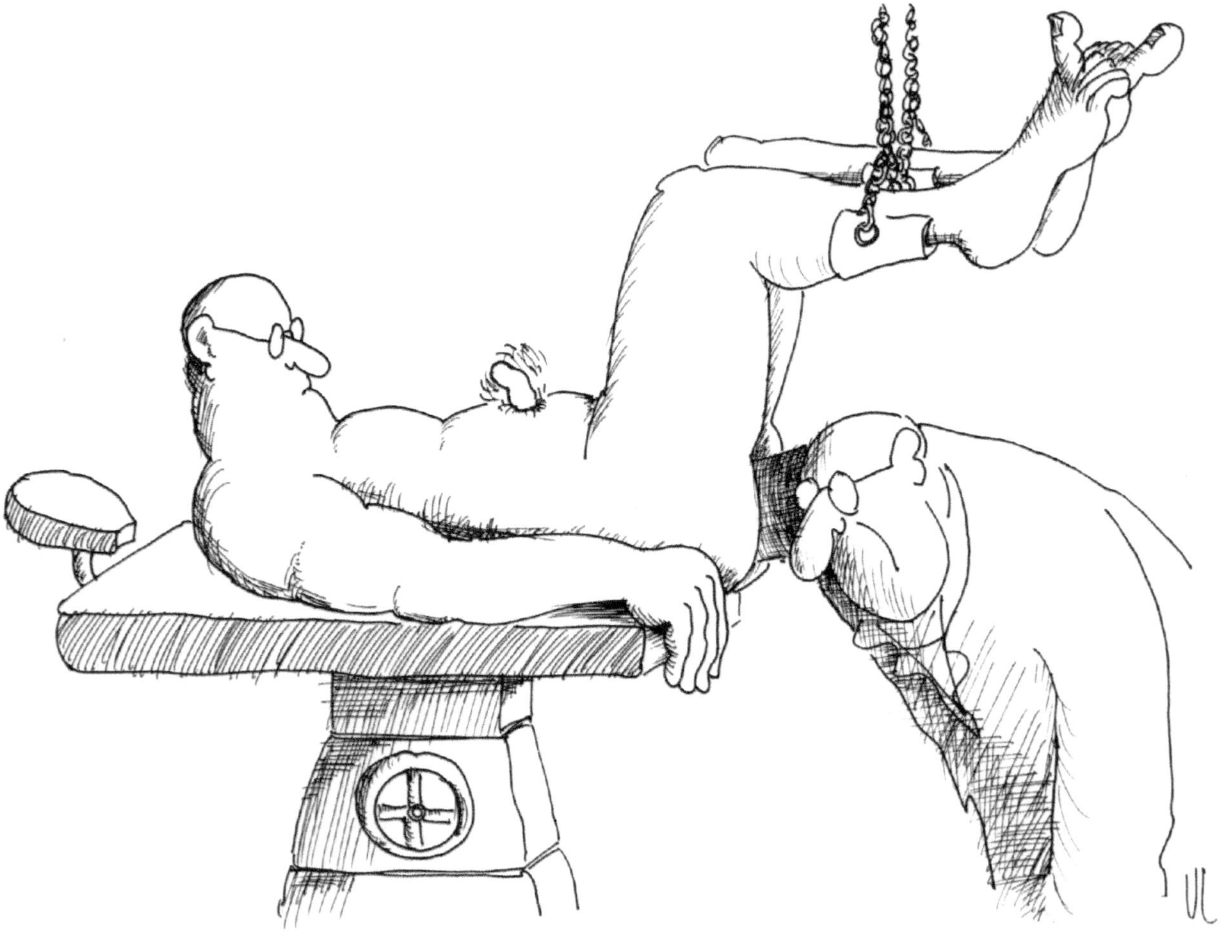

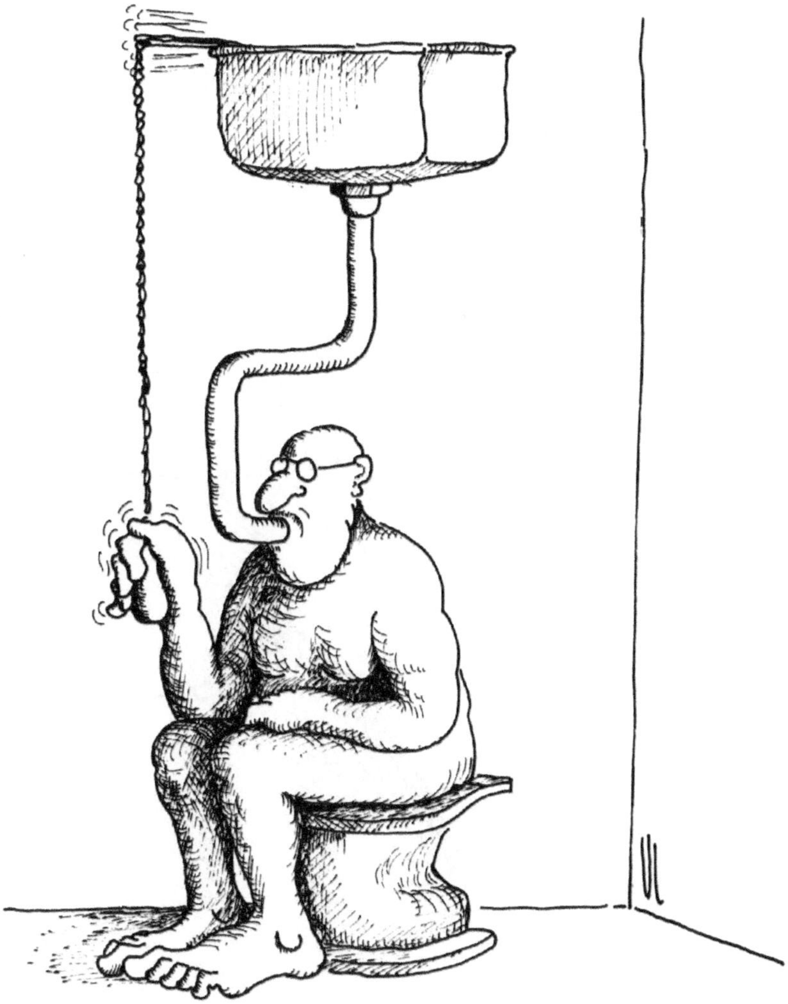

# PSYCHIATRY

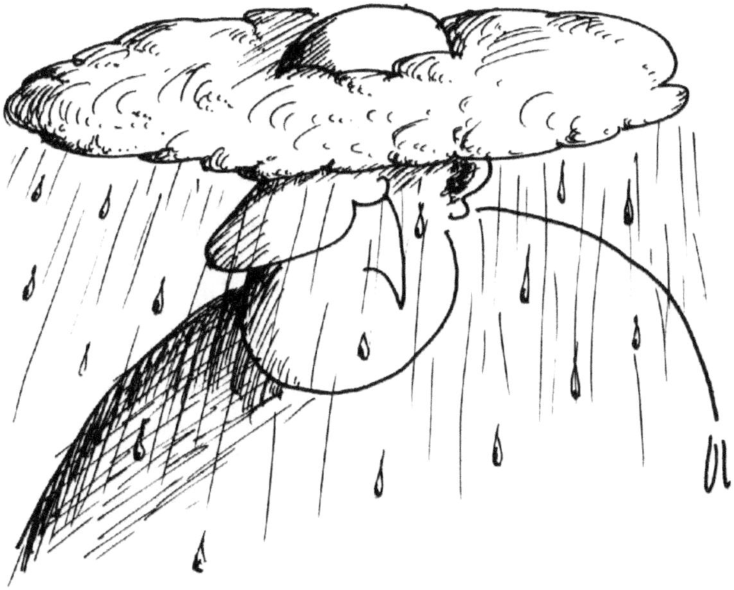

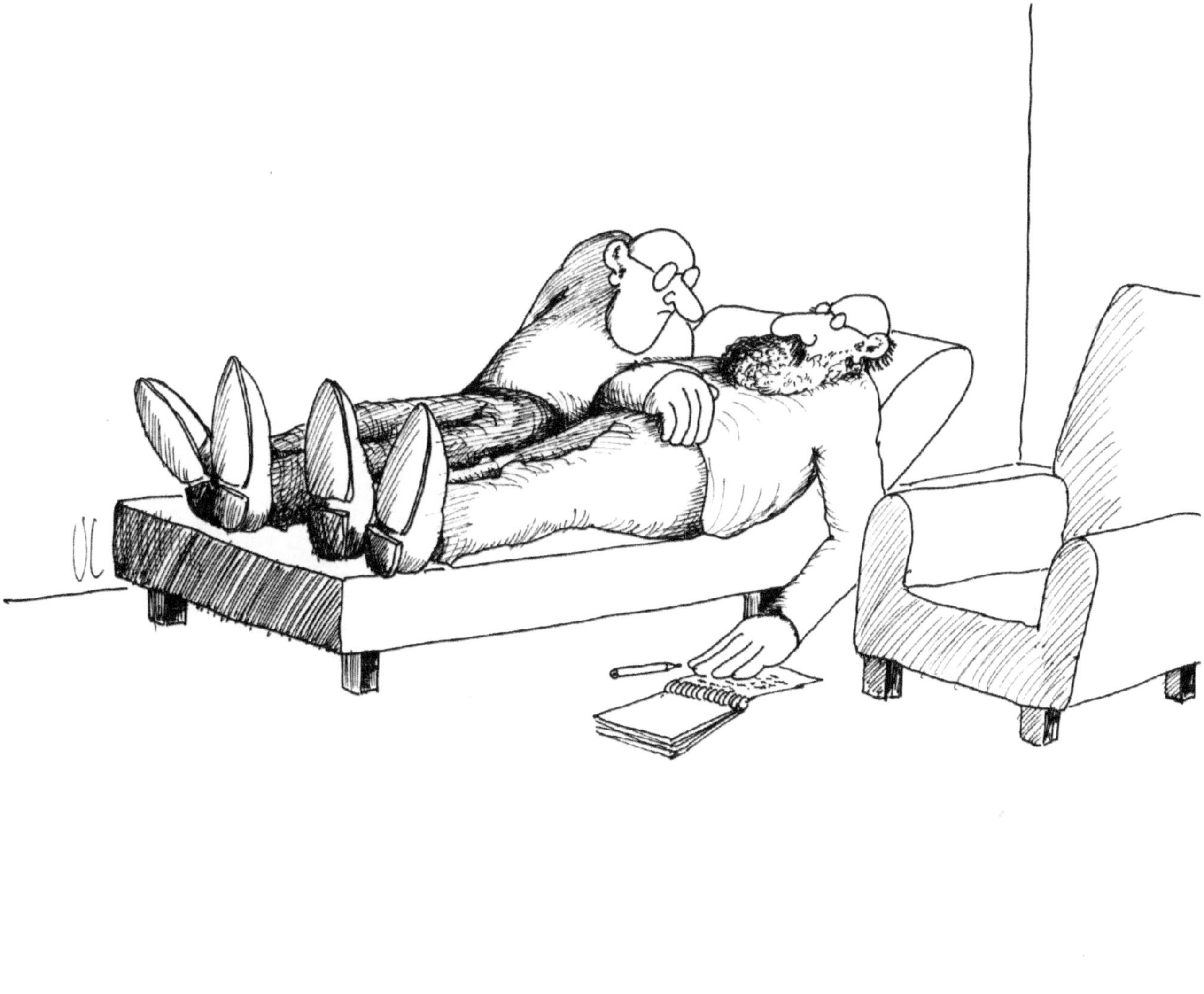

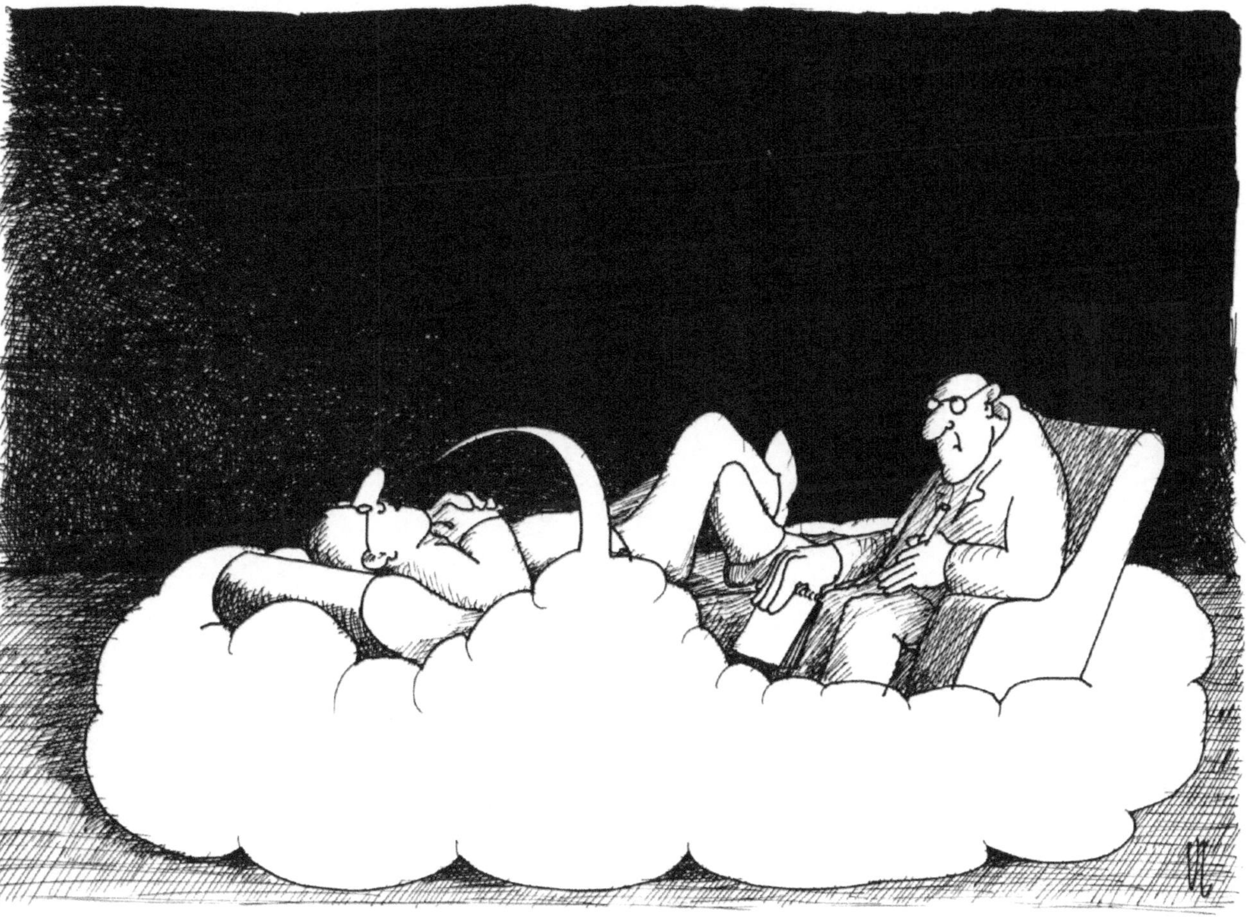

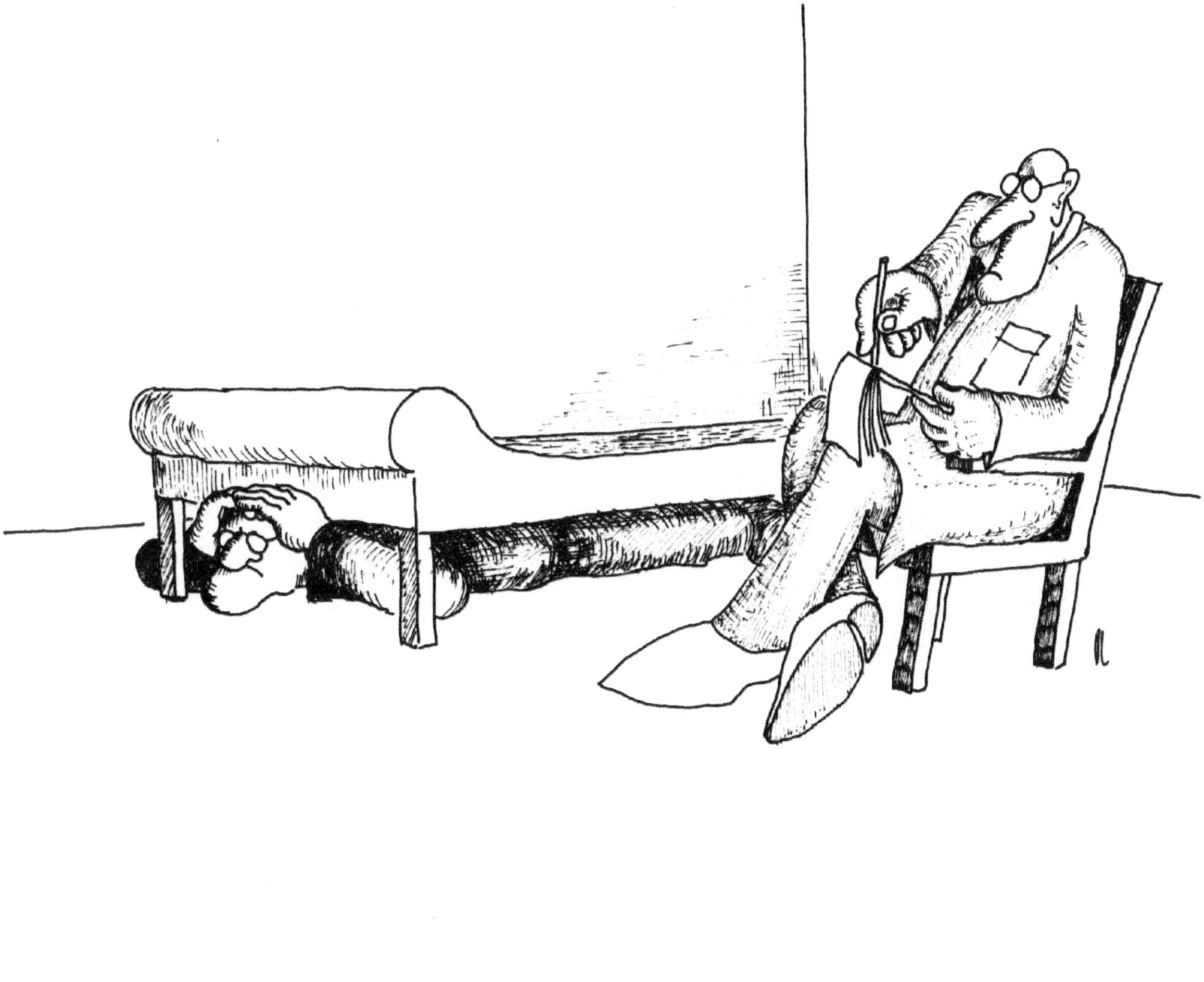

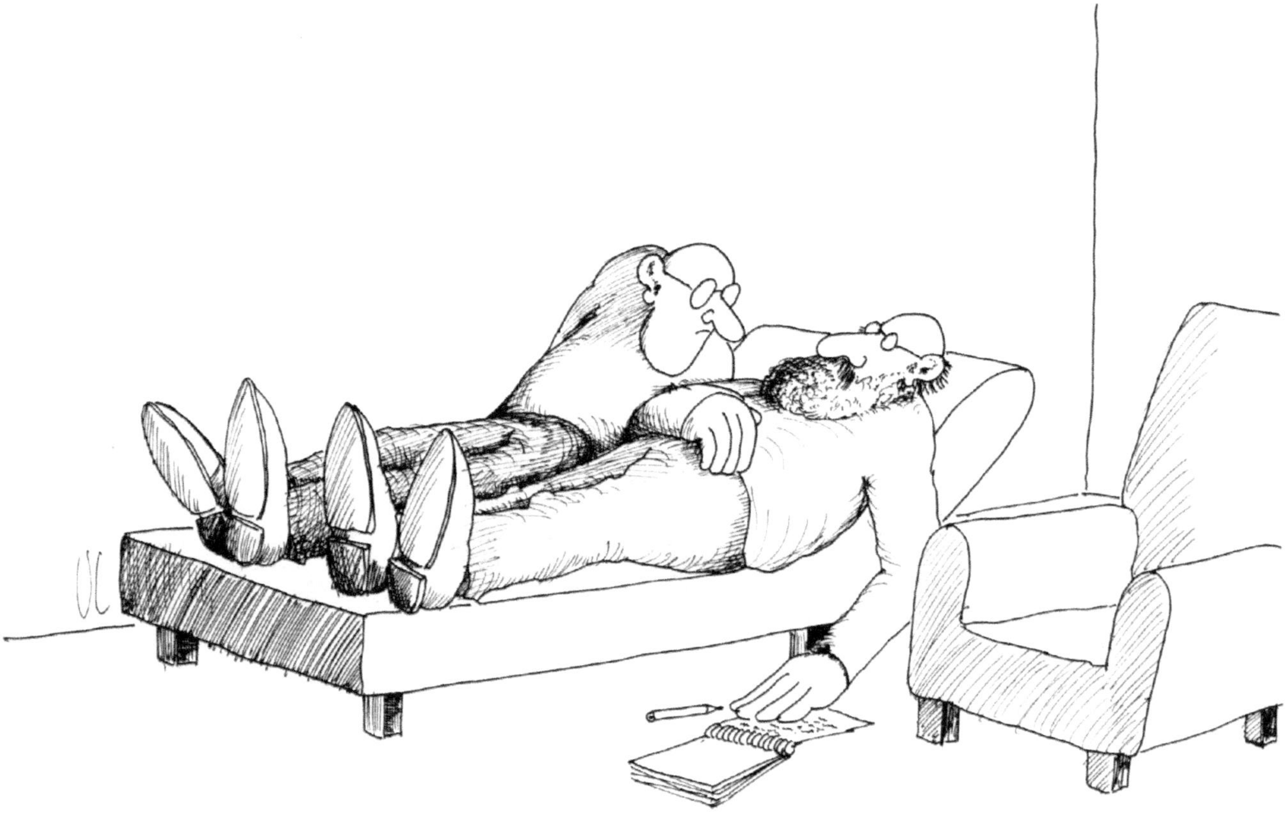

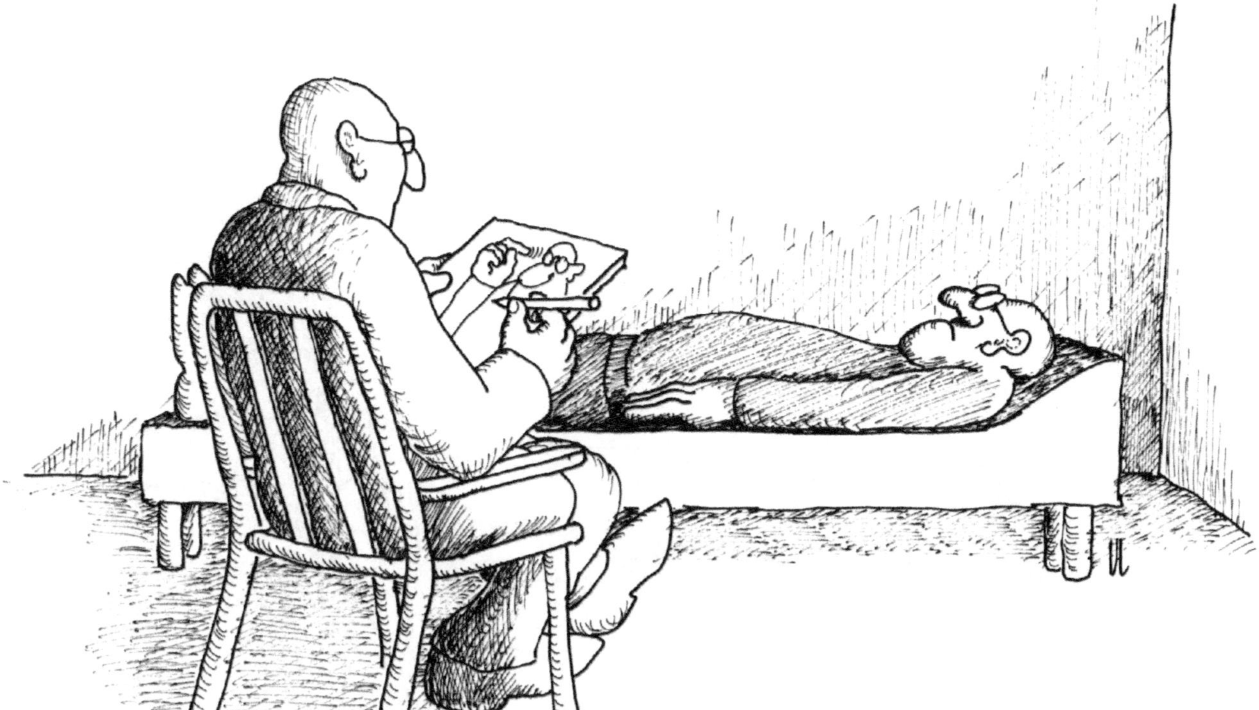

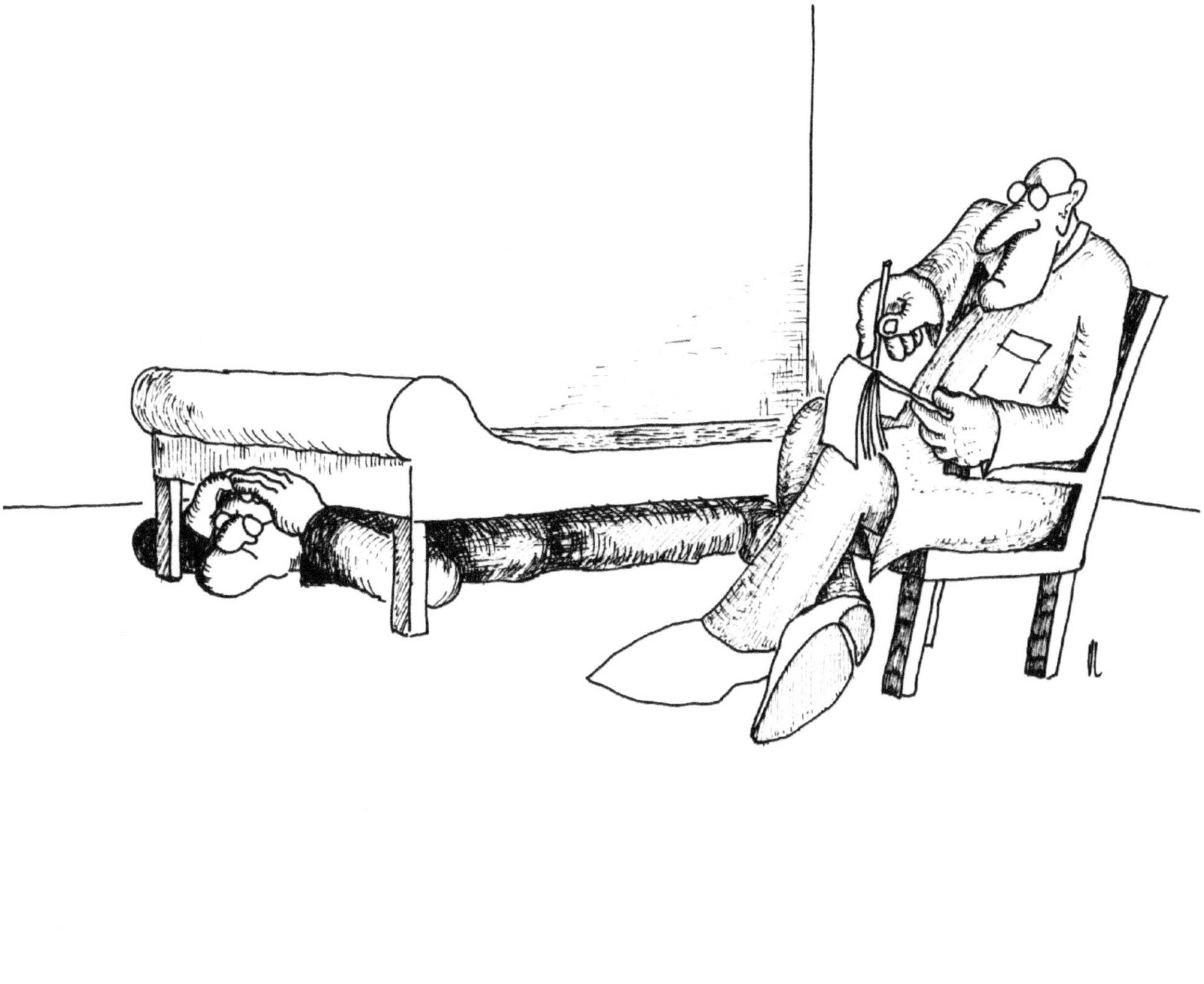

# RADIOLOGY

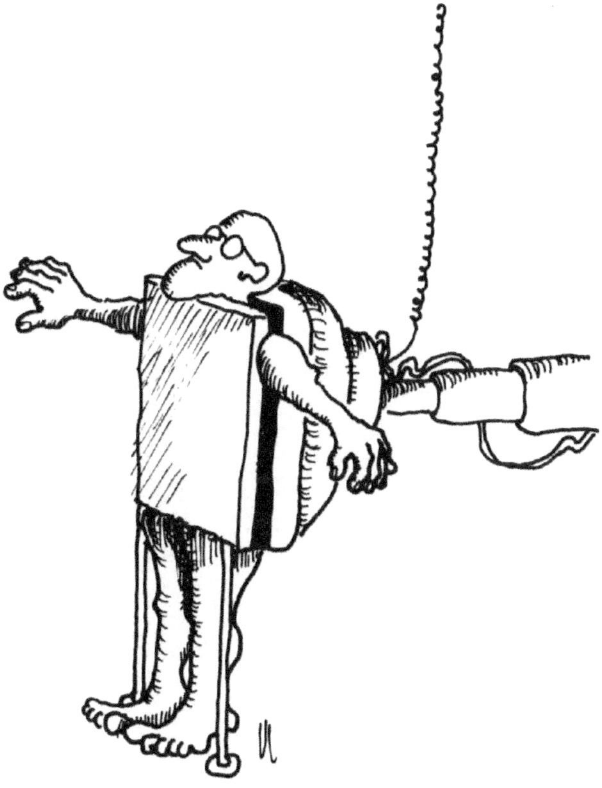

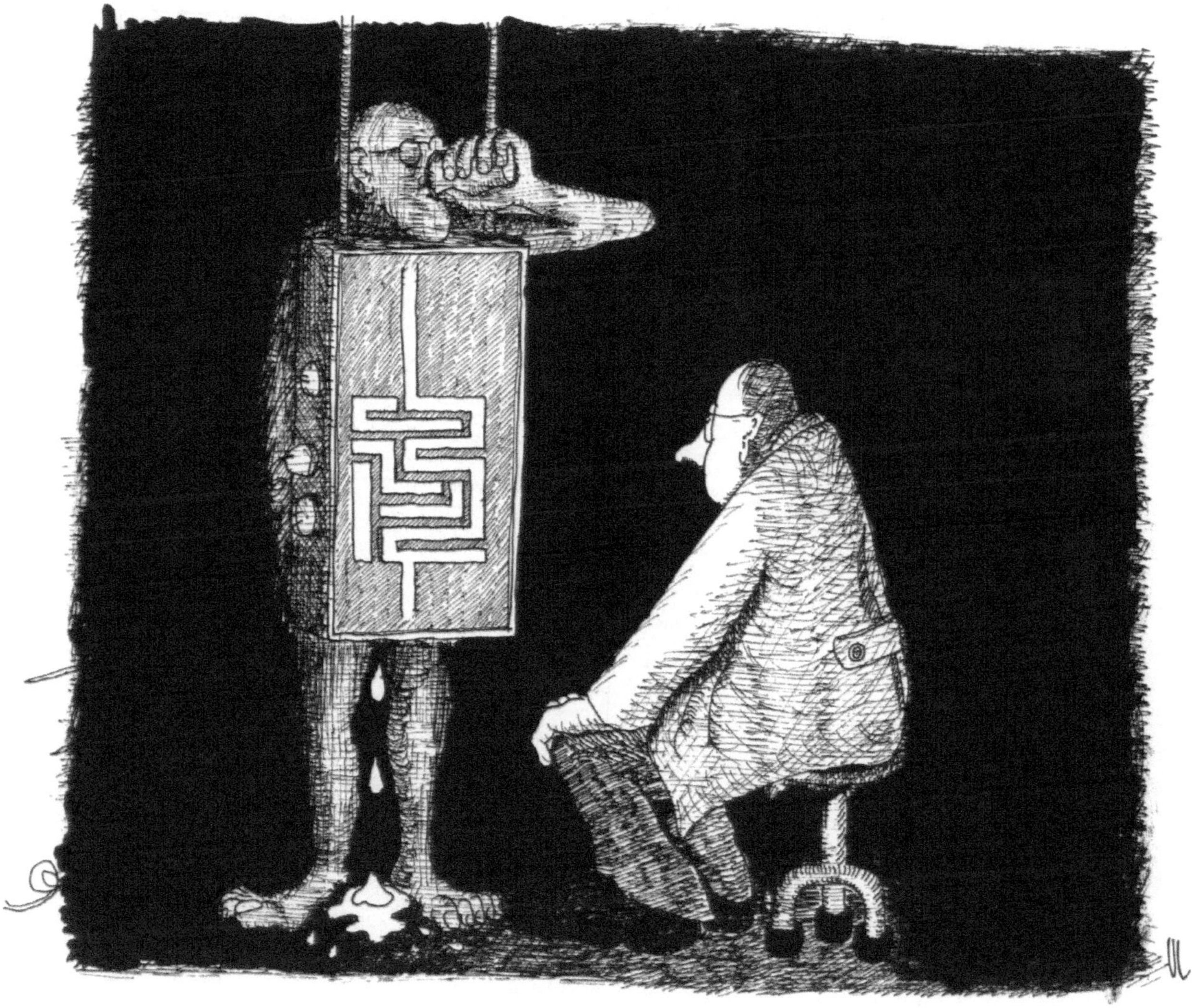

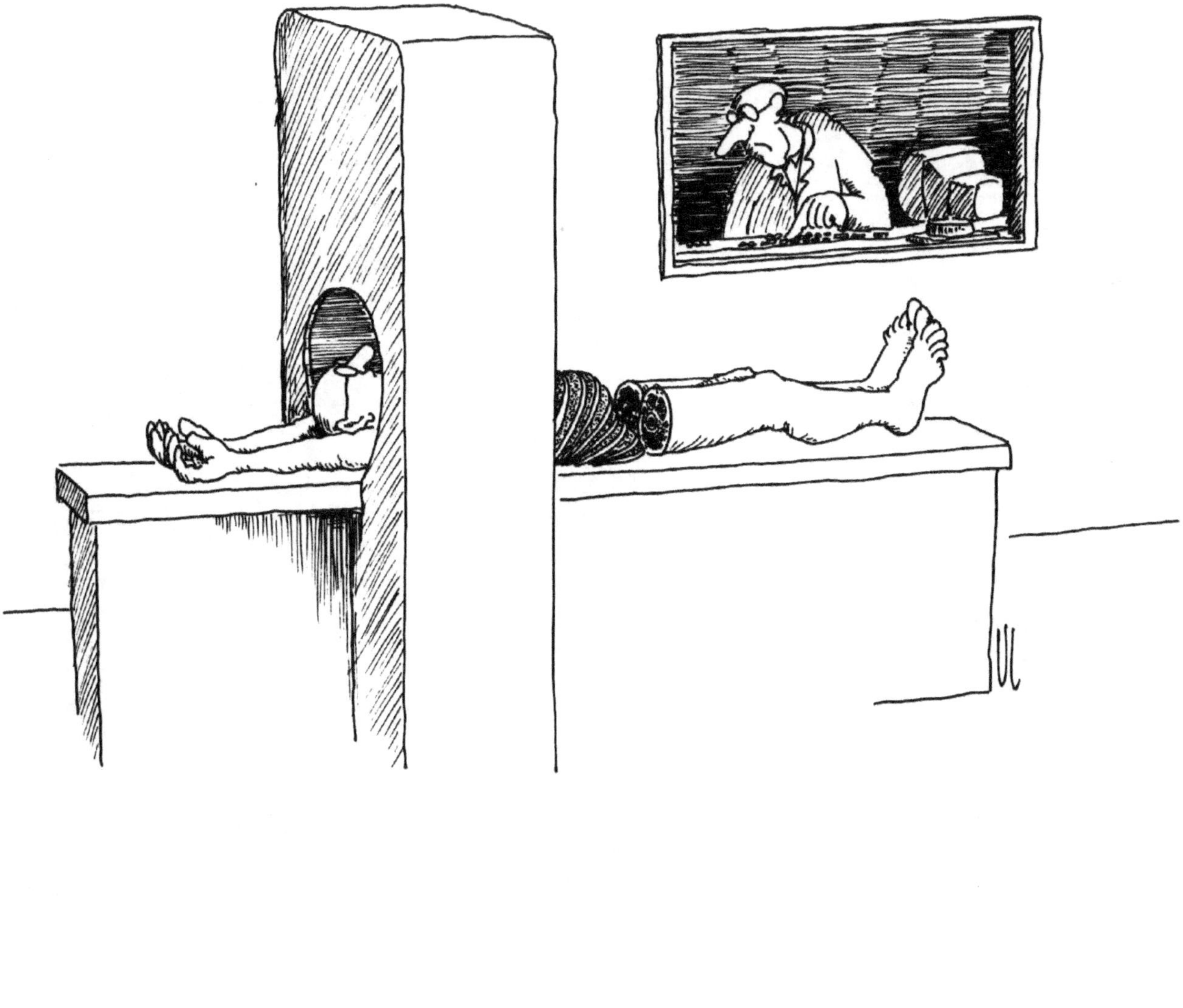

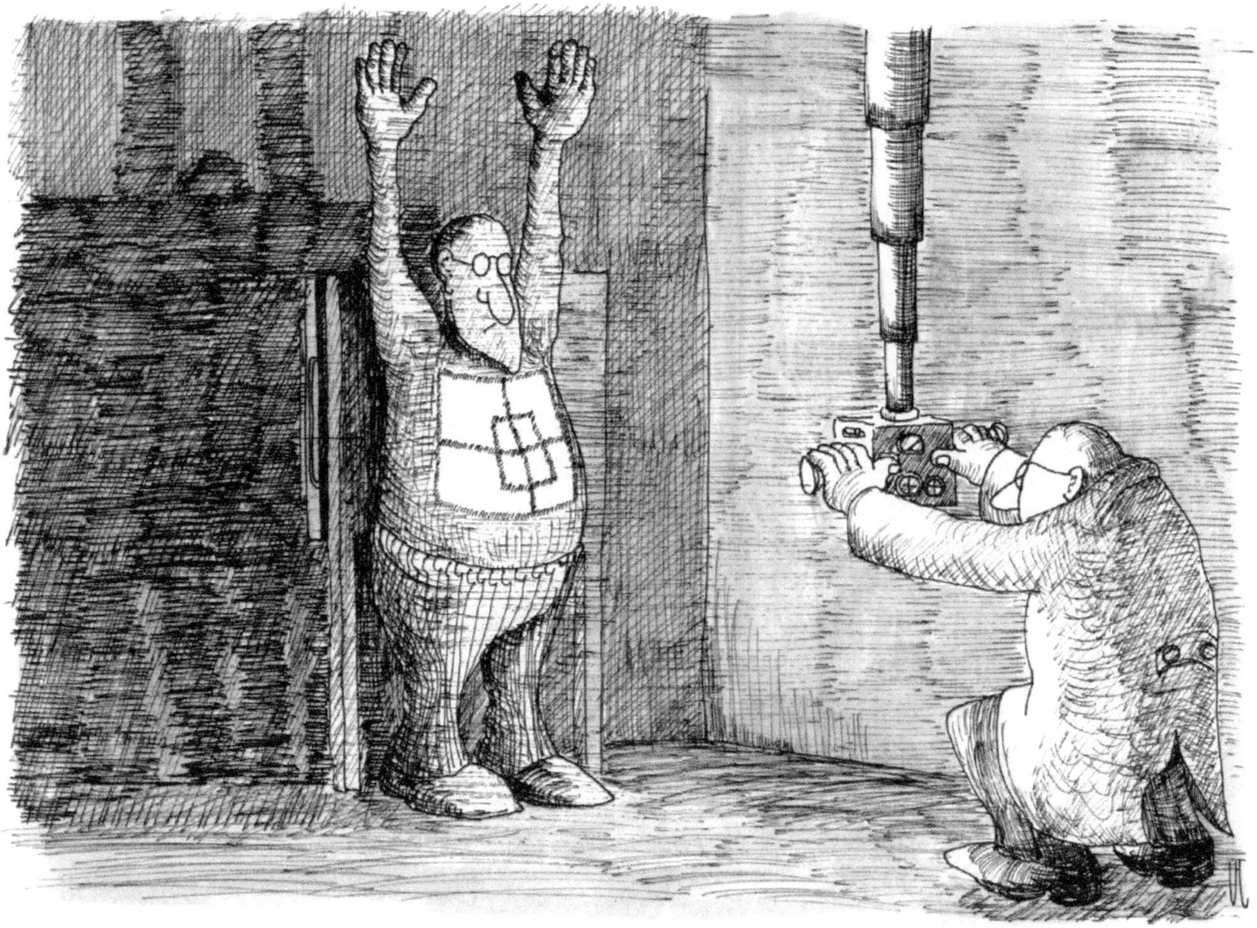

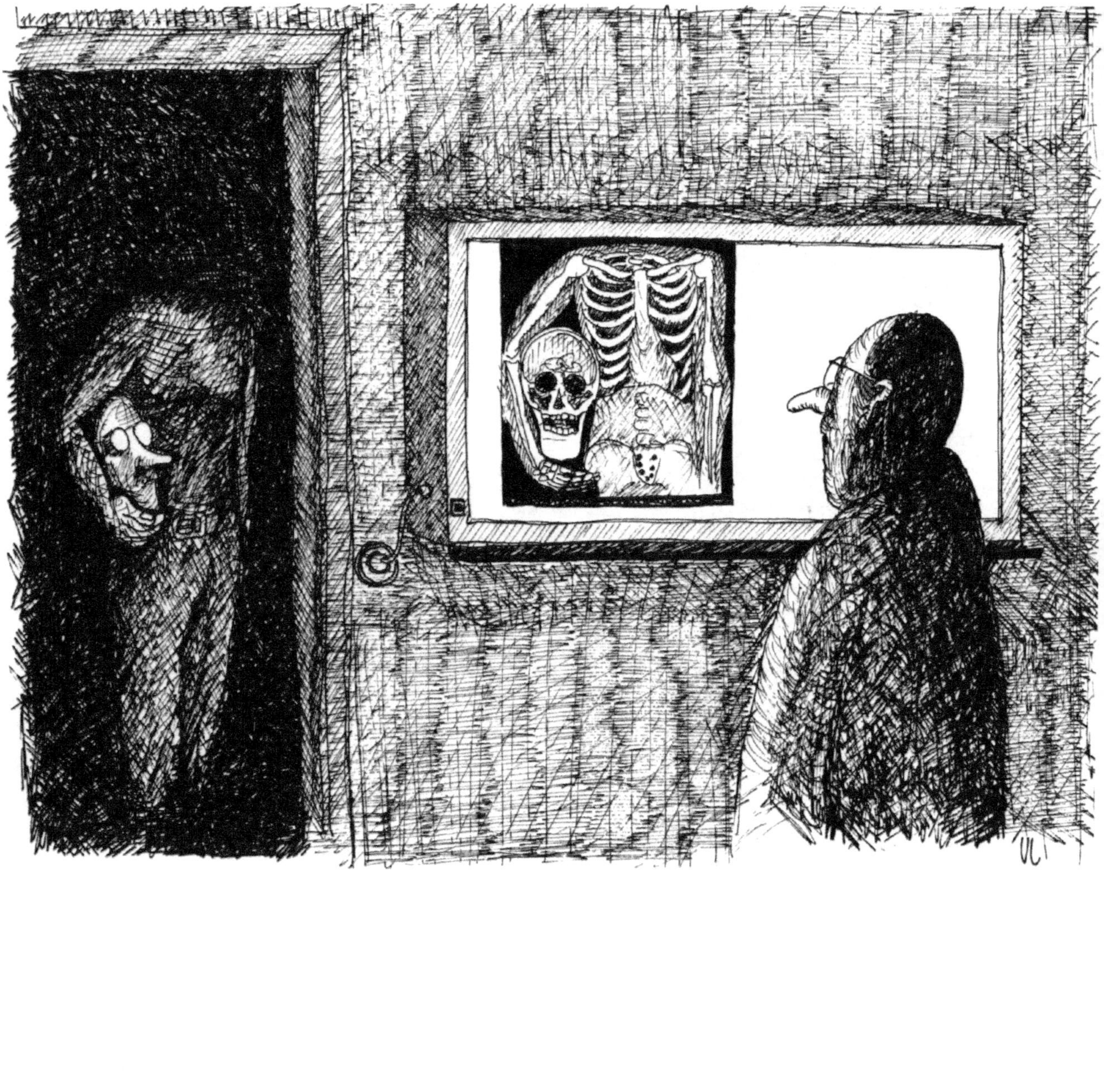

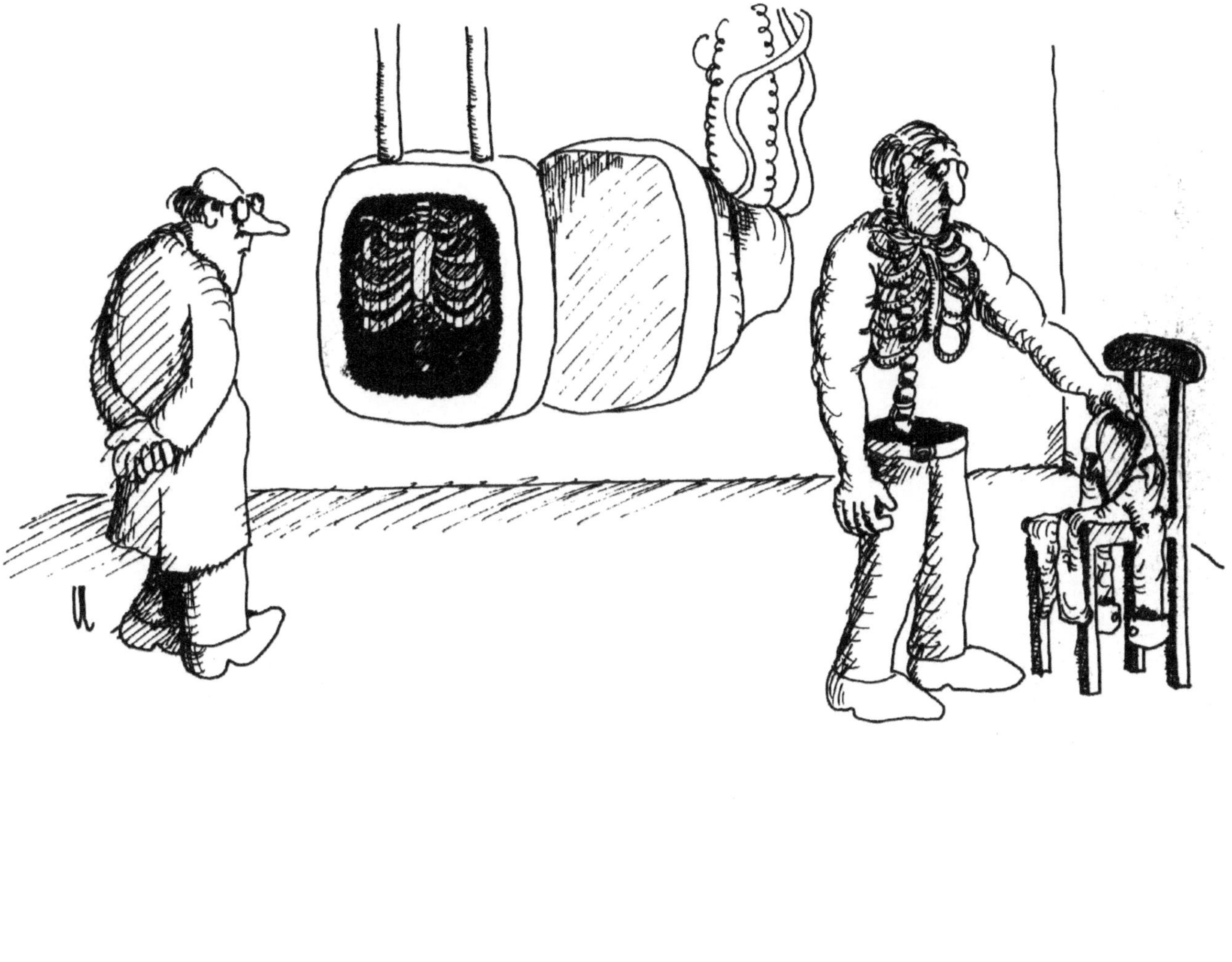

# SEXUAL MEDICINE

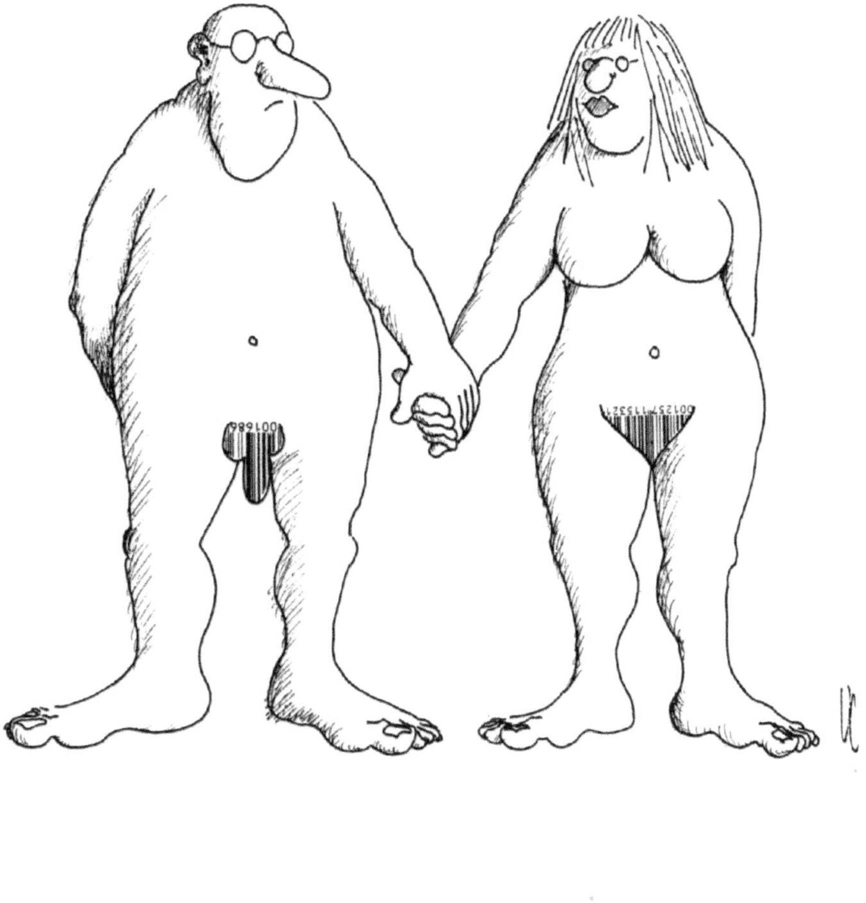

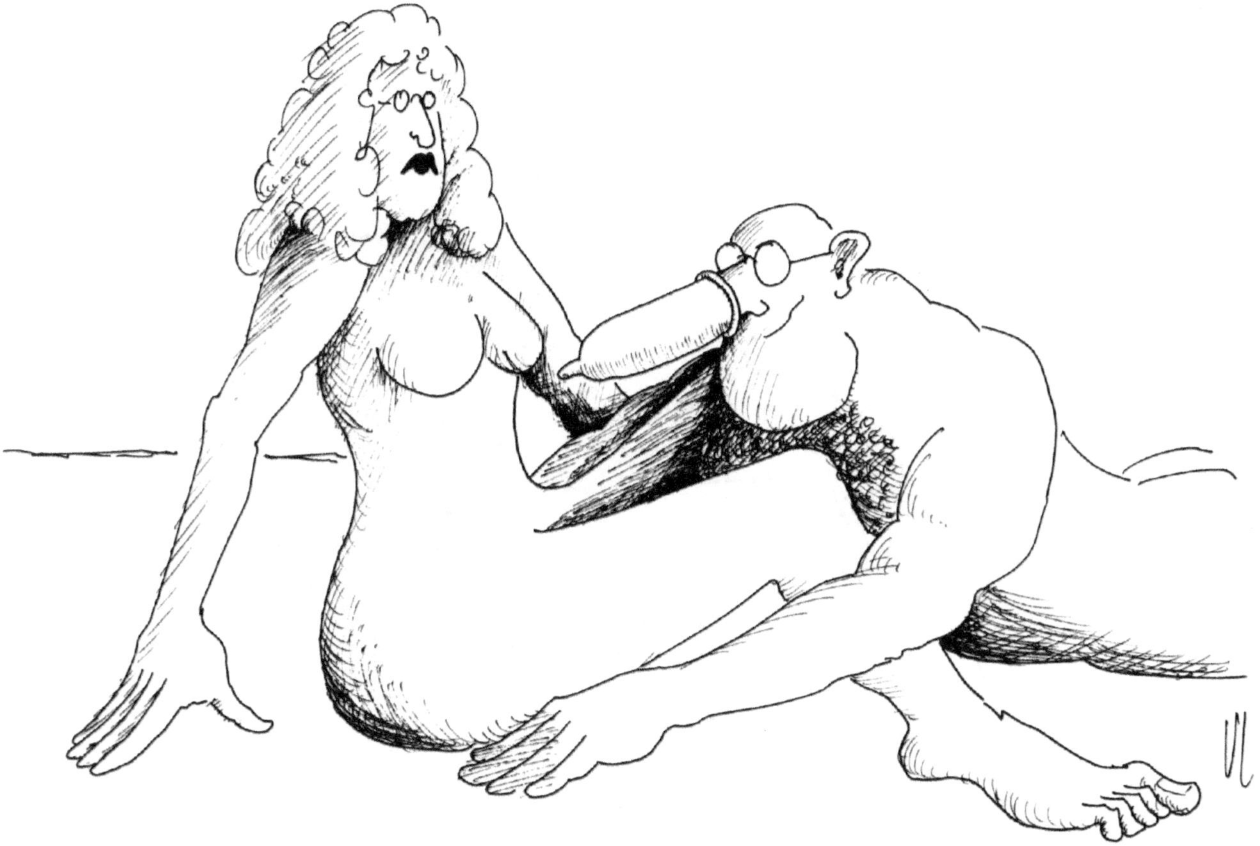

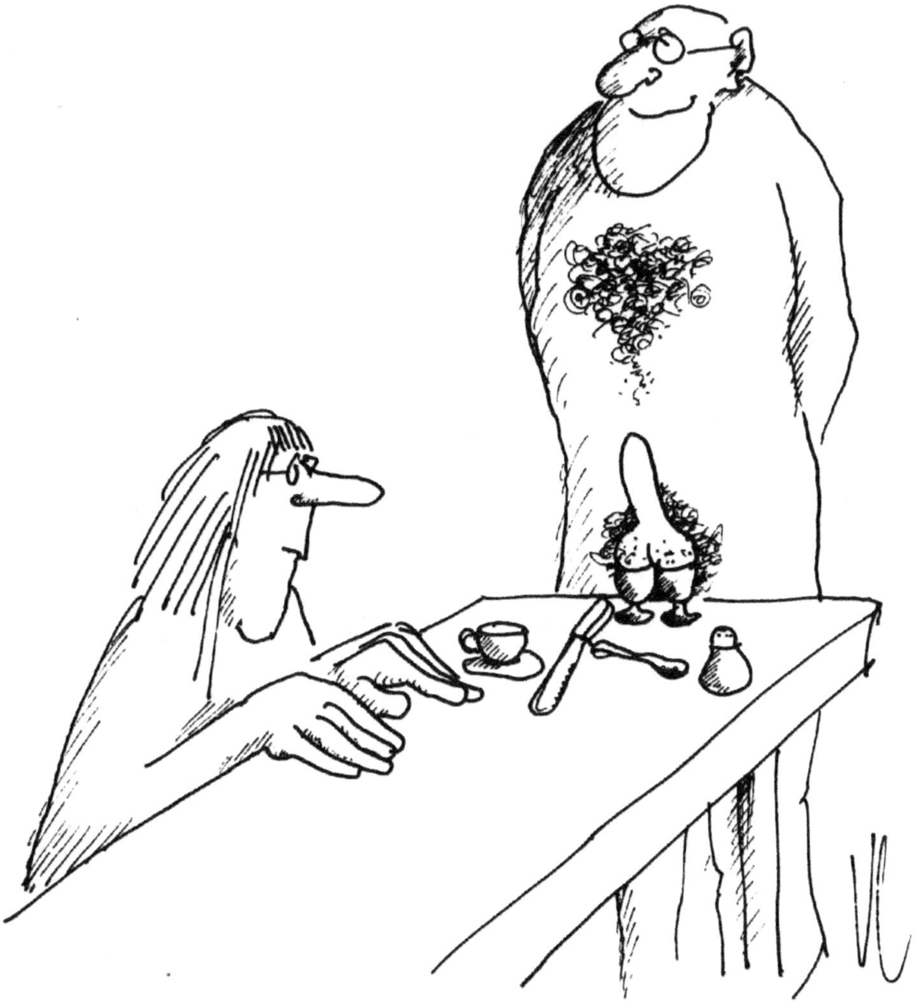

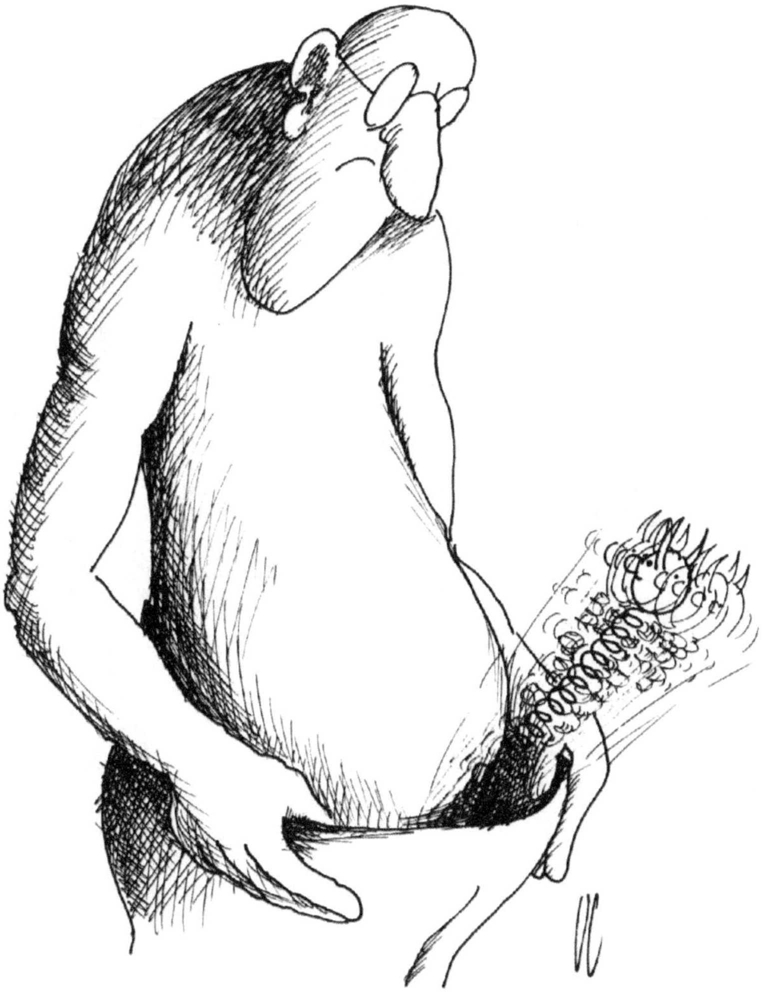

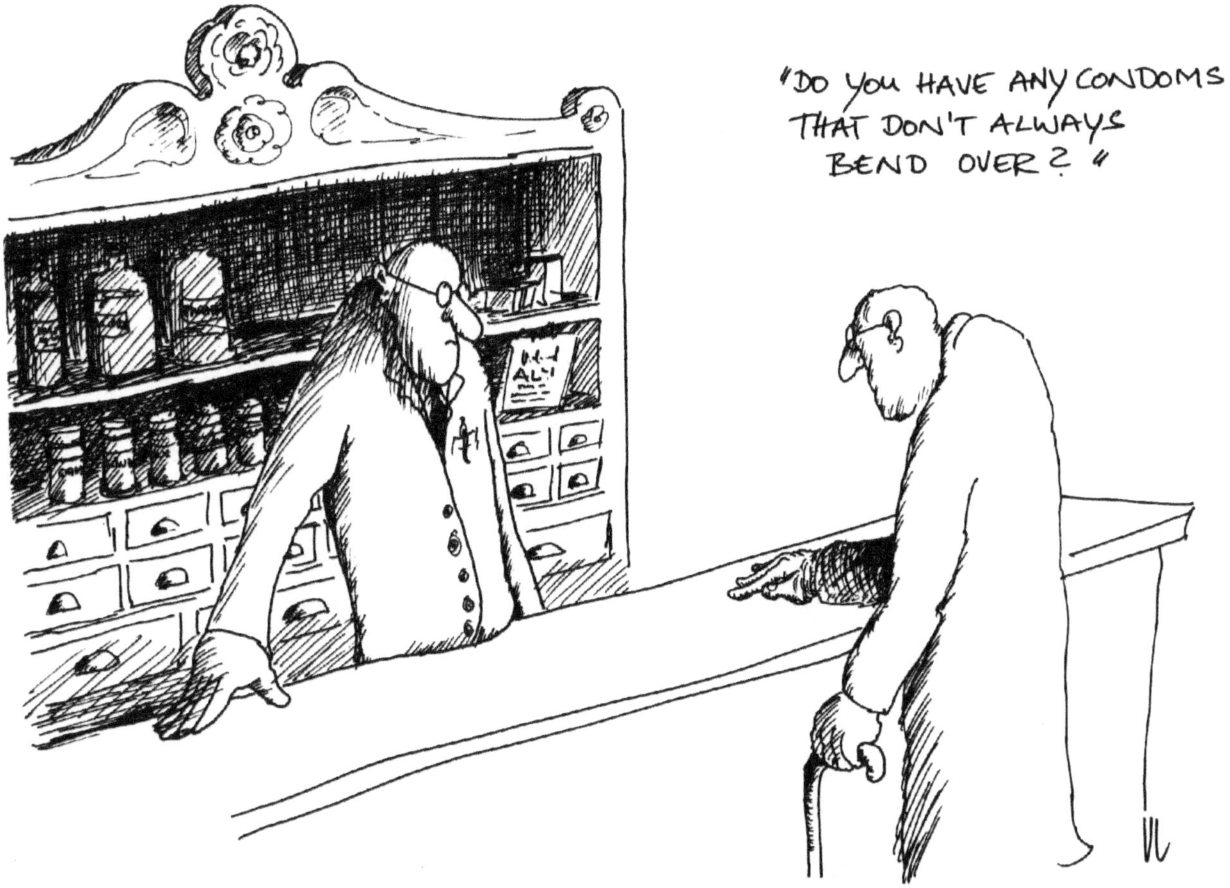
"DO YOU HAVE ANY CONDOMS THAT DON'T ALWAYS BEND OVER?"

# TRAUMA-TOLOGY

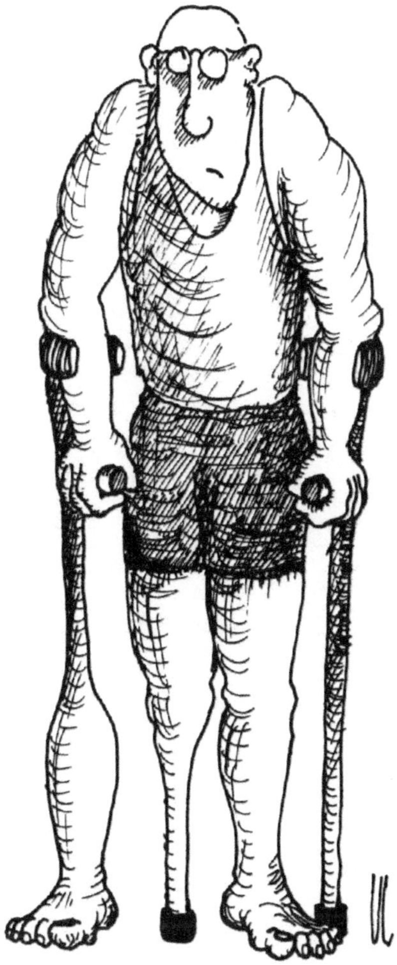

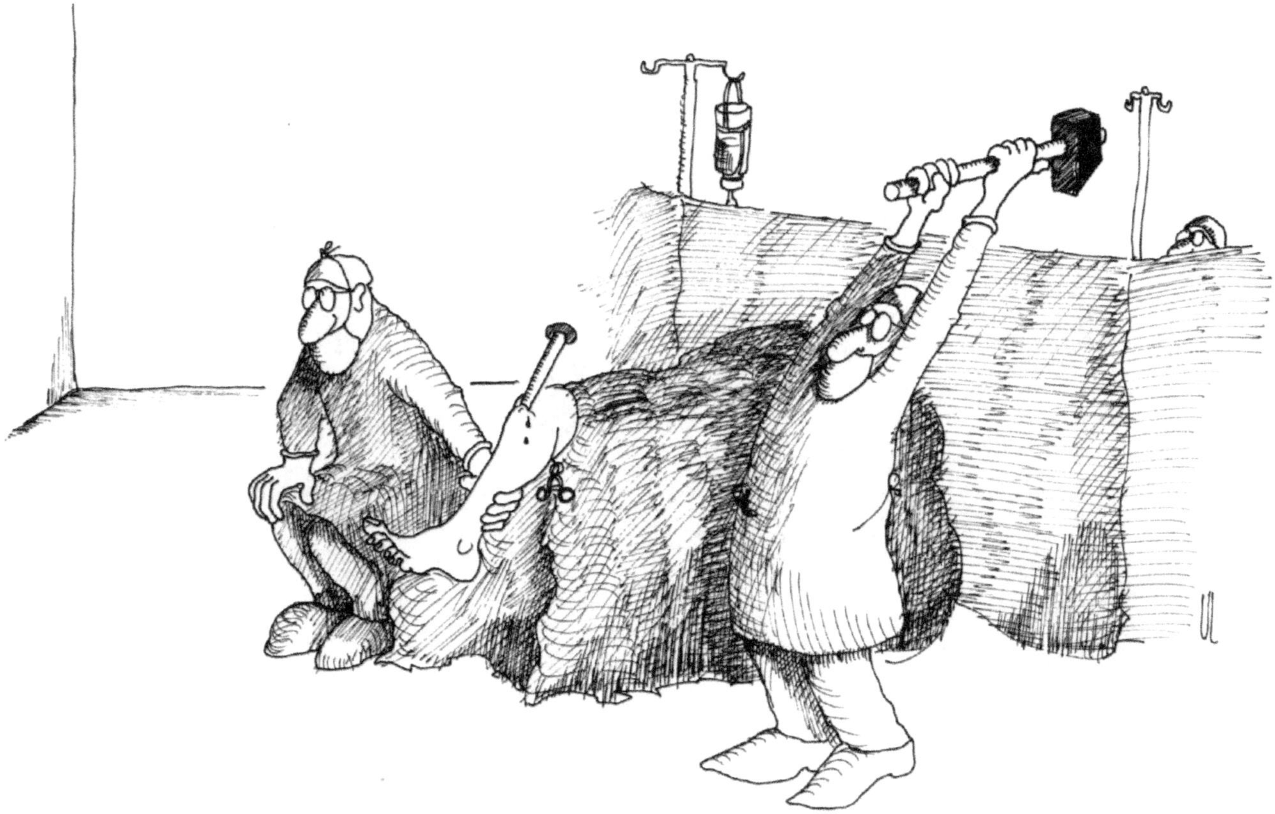

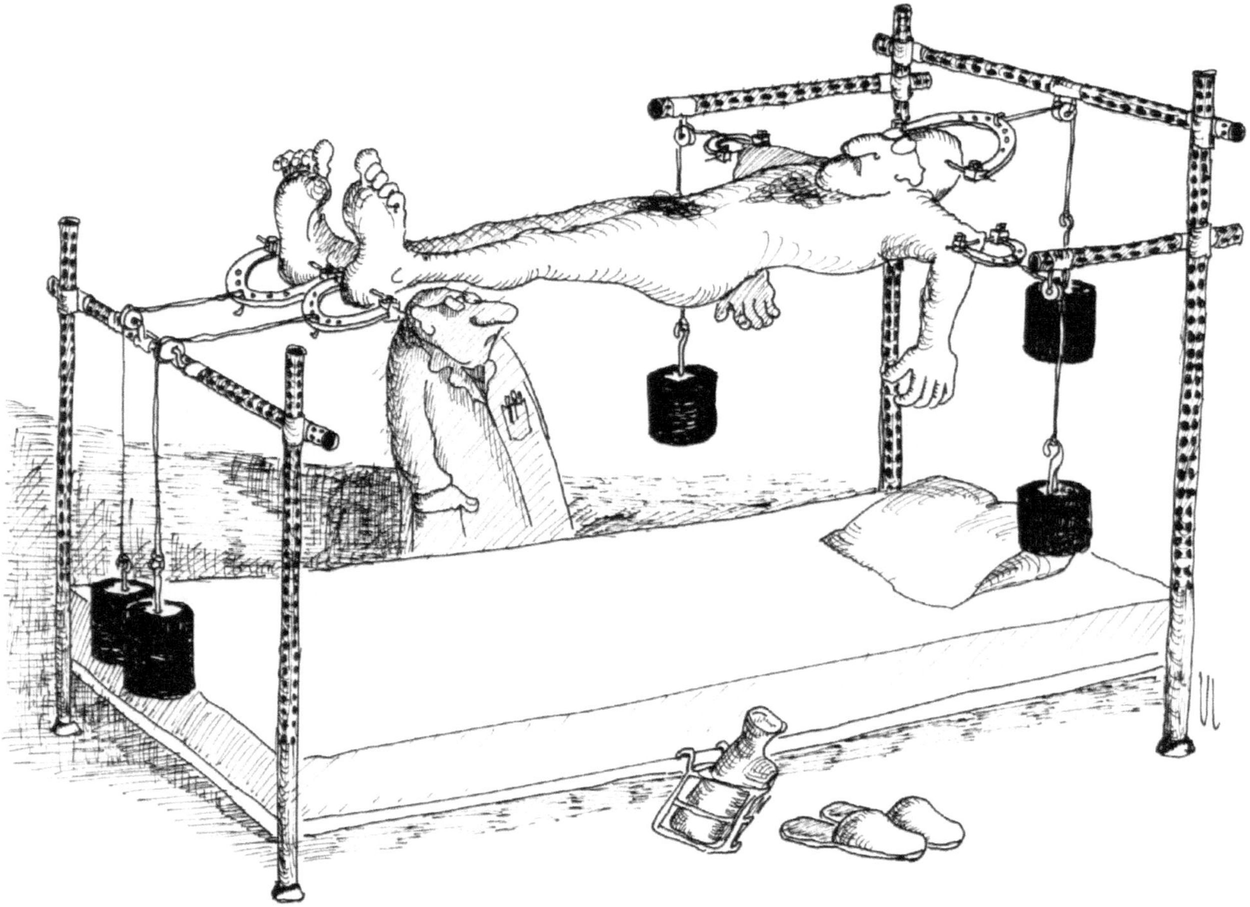

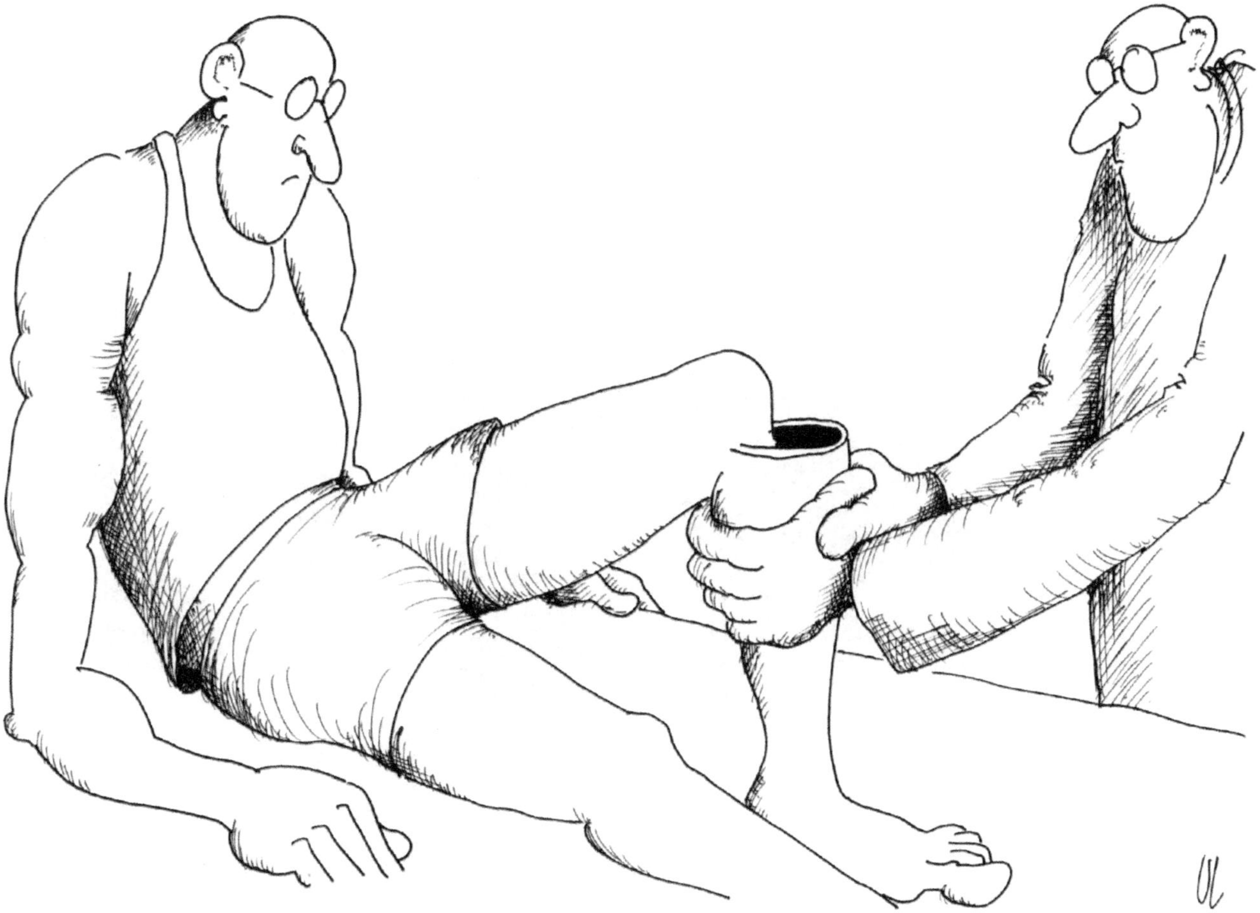

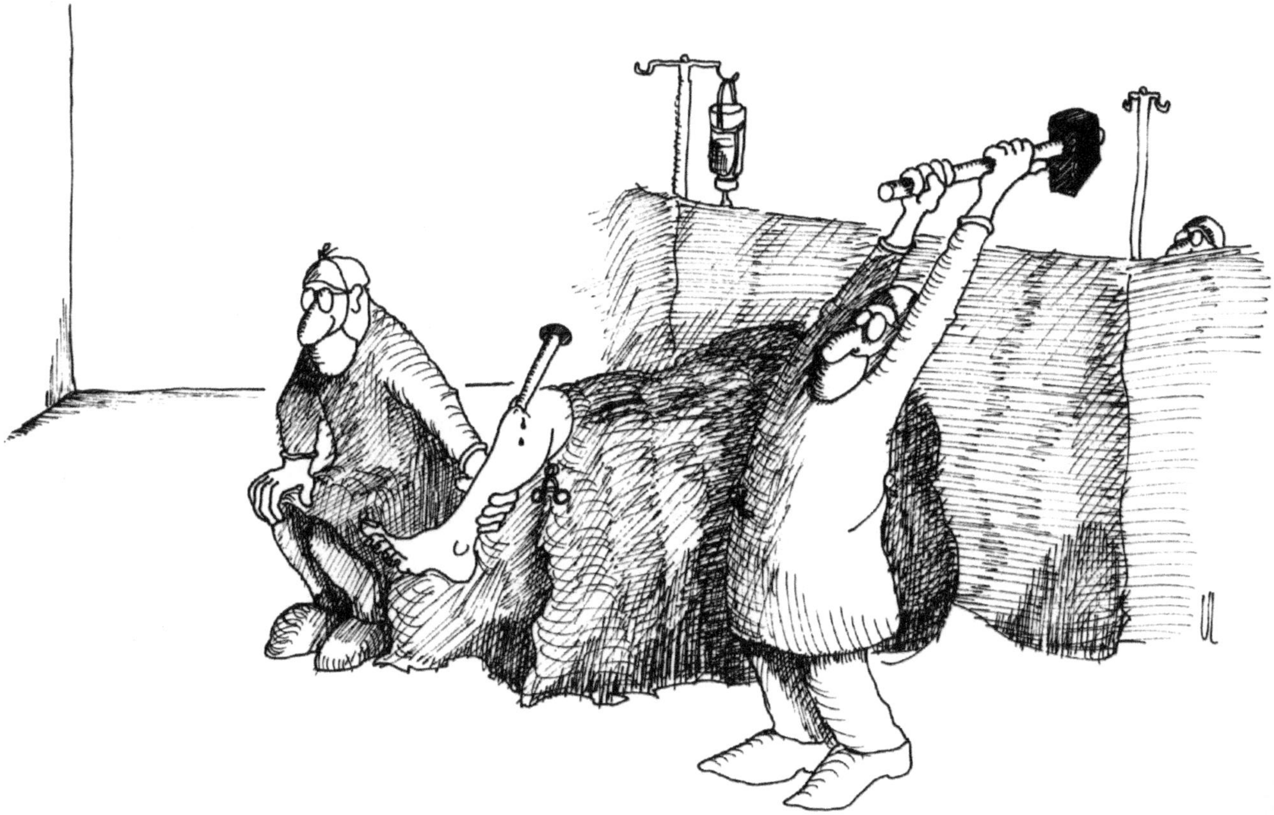

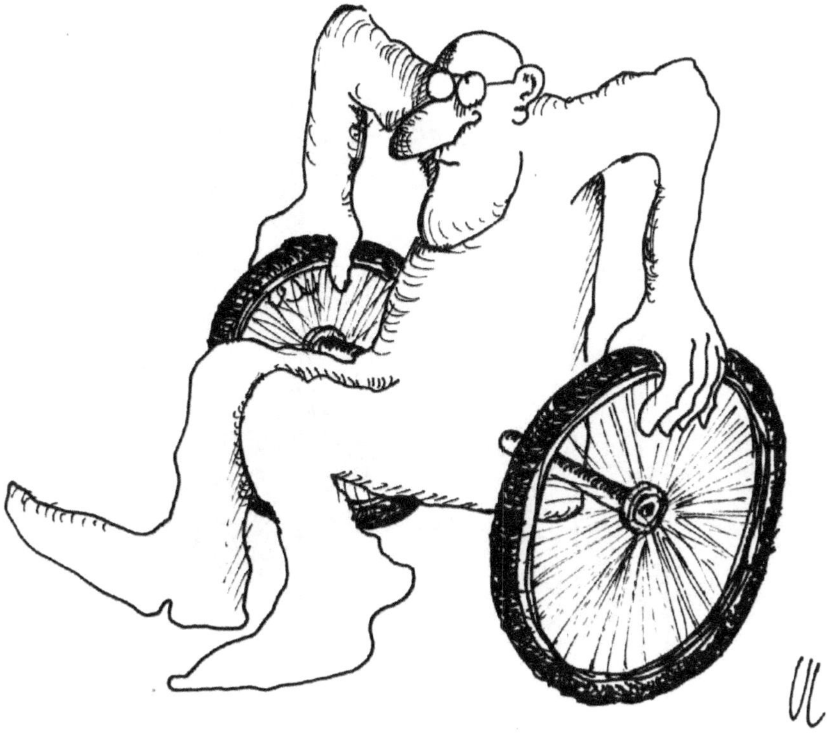

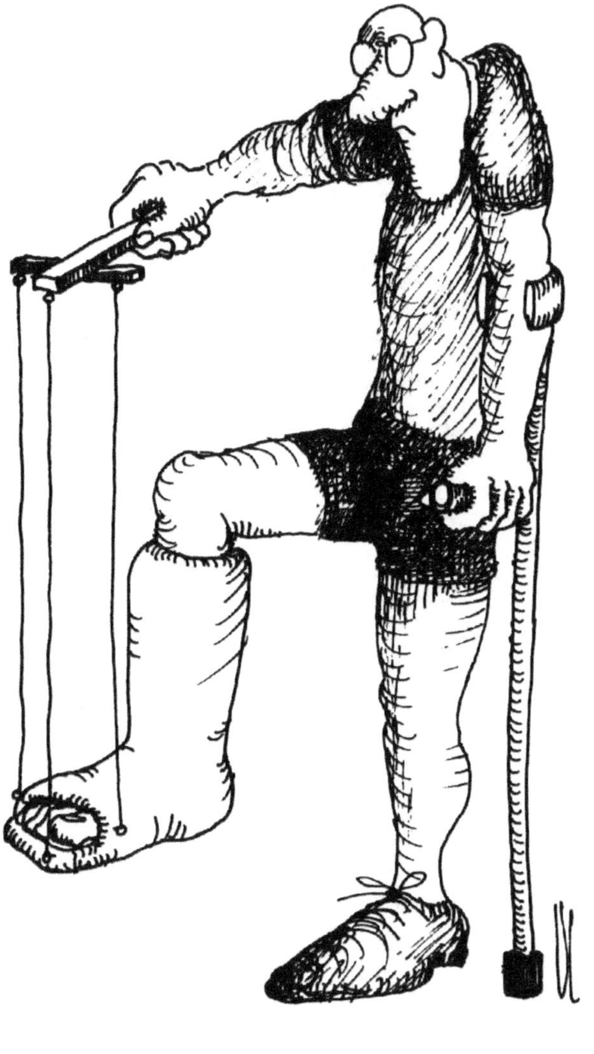

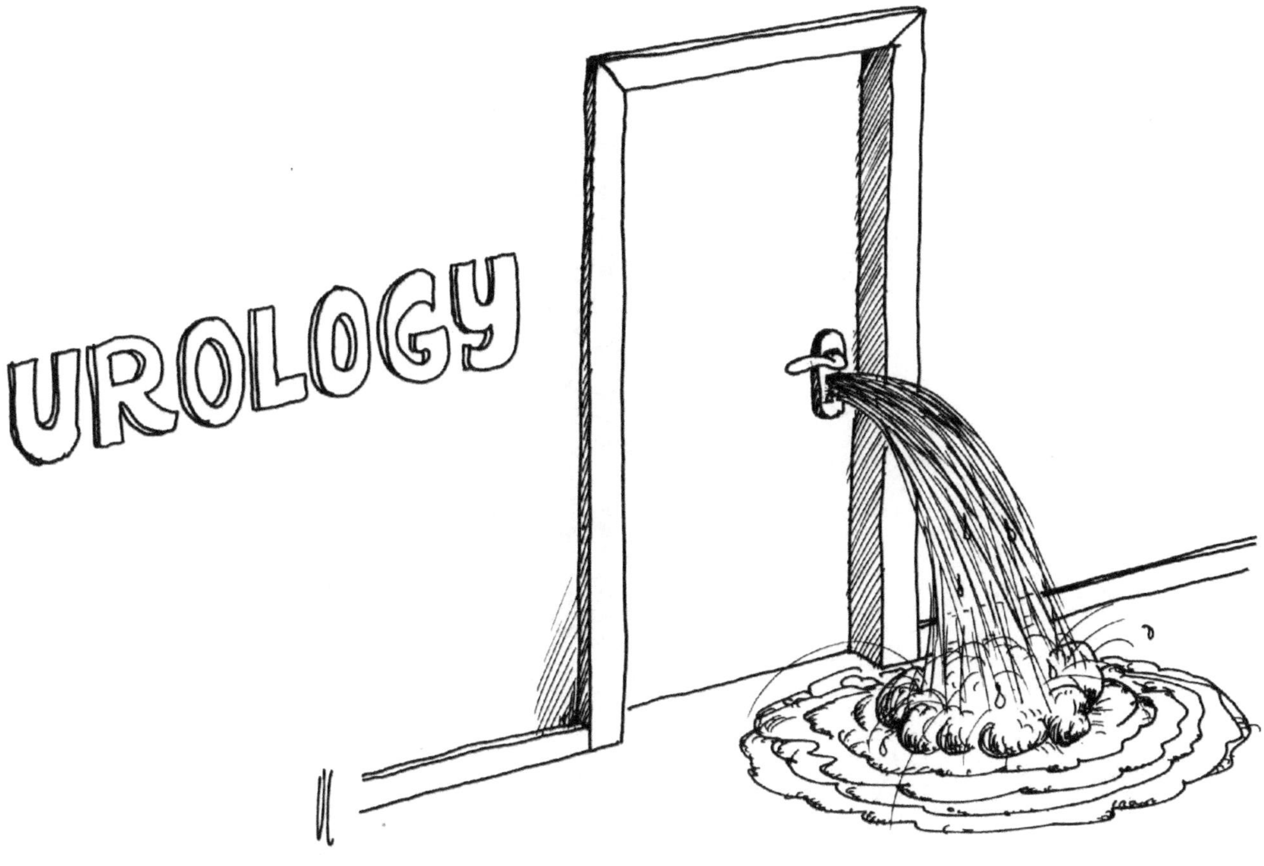
UROLOGY

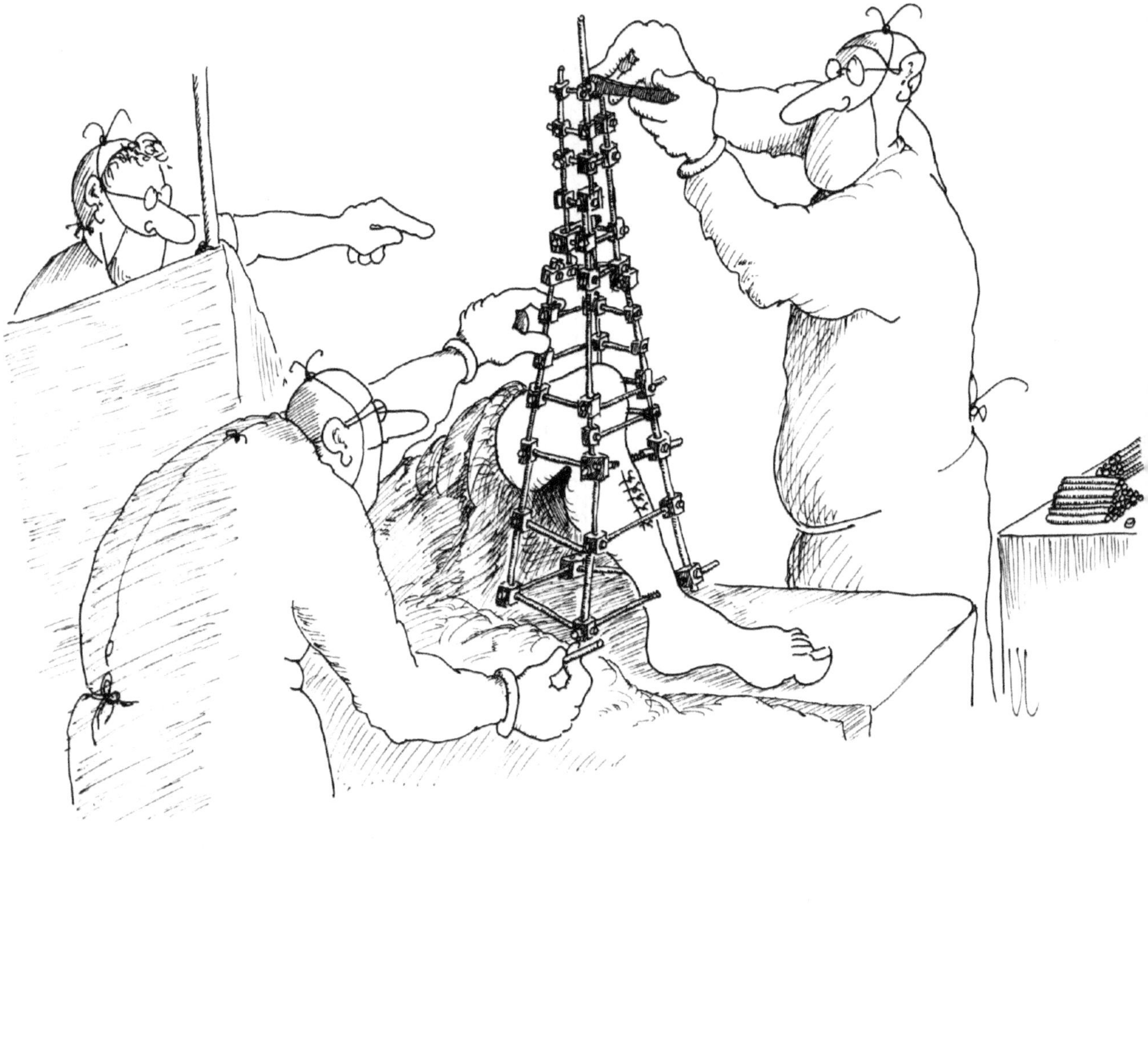

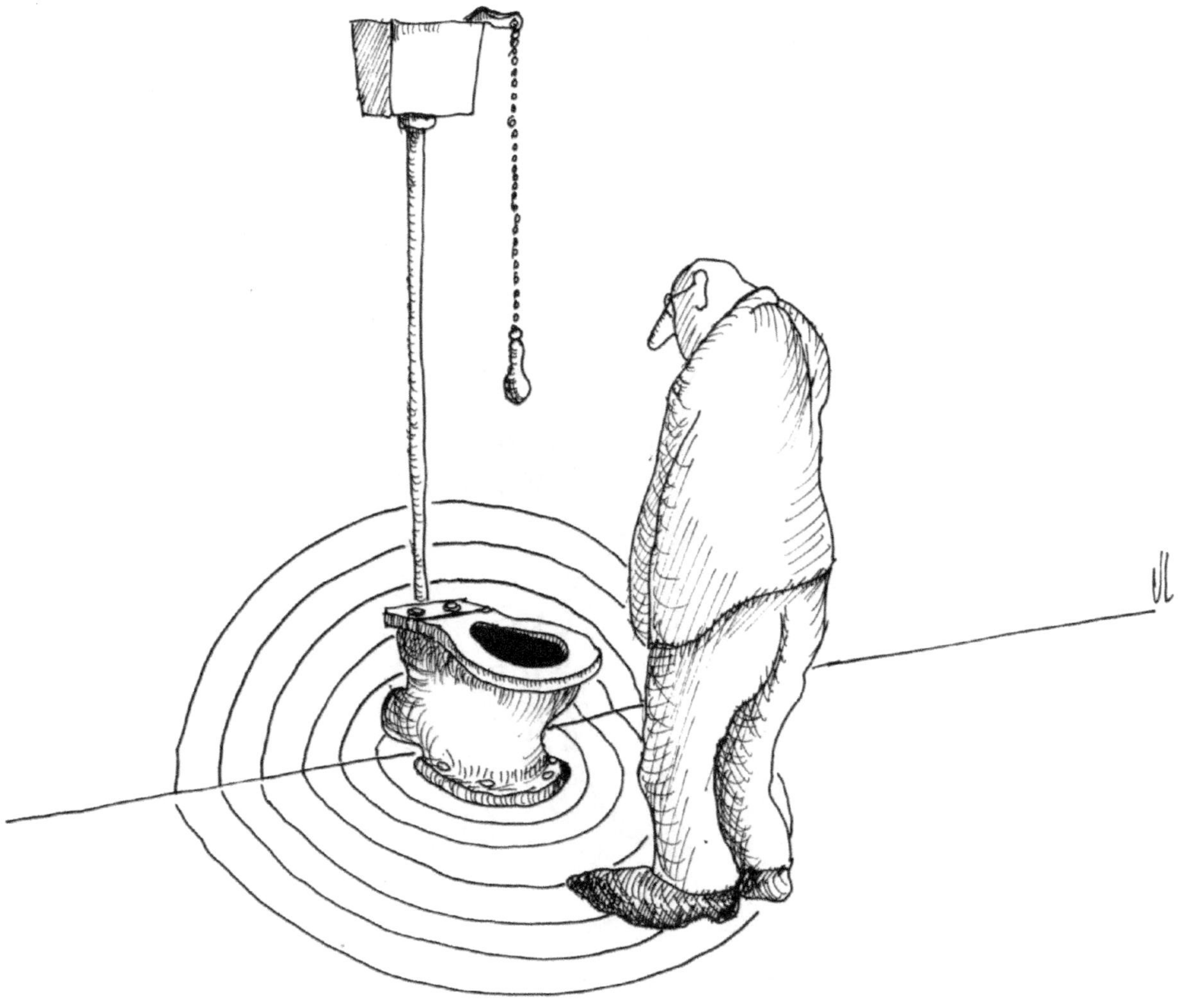

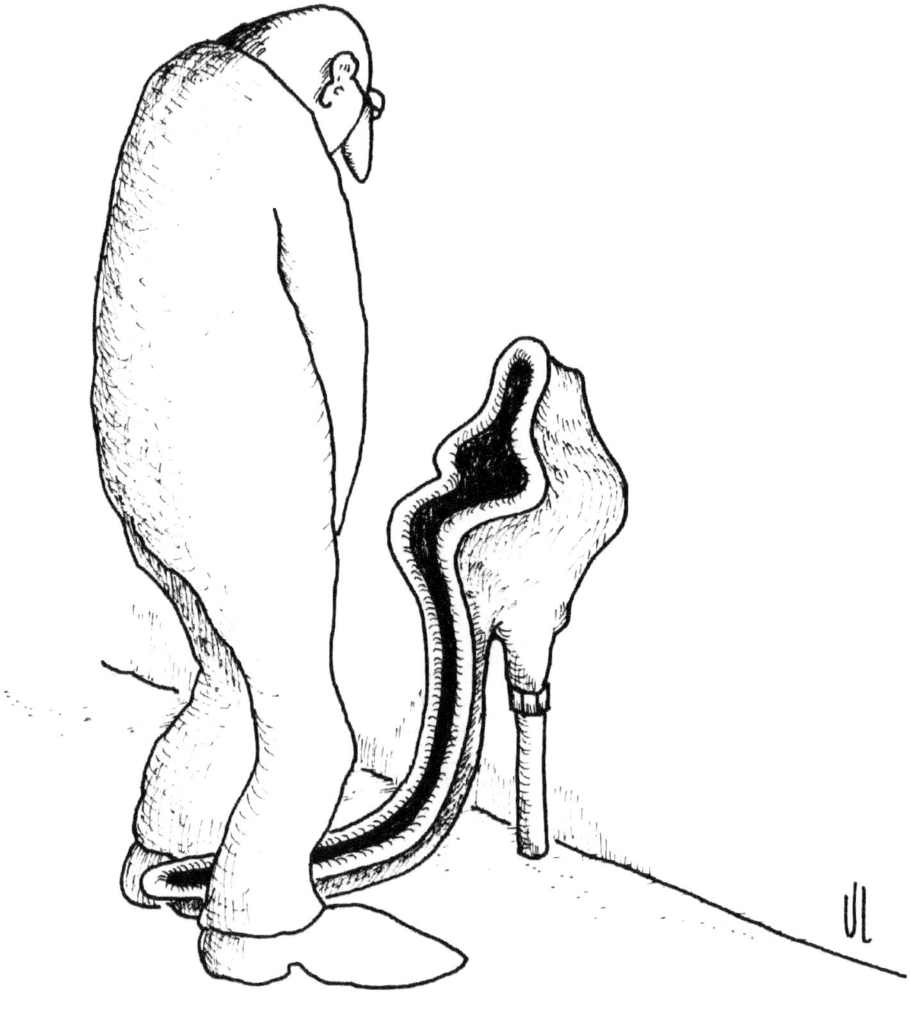

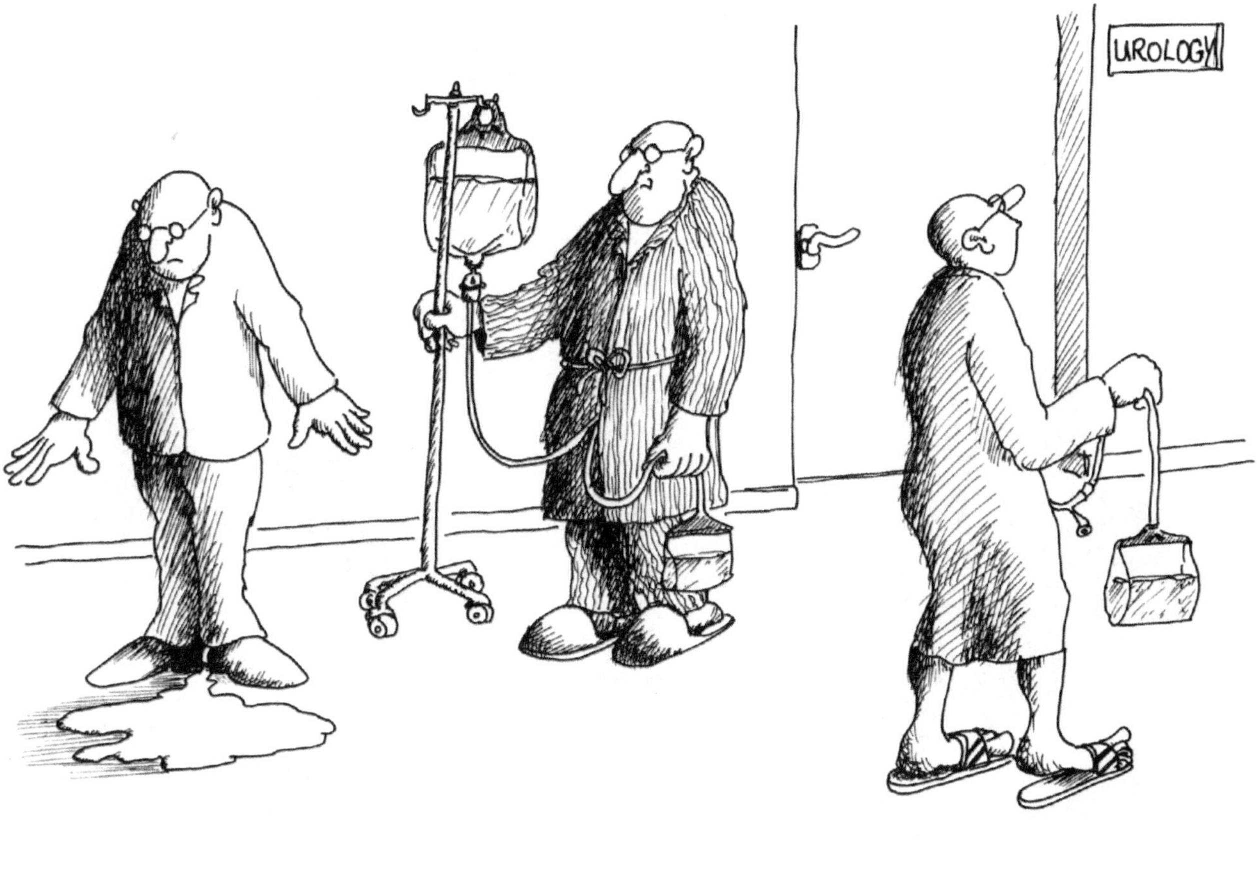
UROLOGY

# DENTISTRY

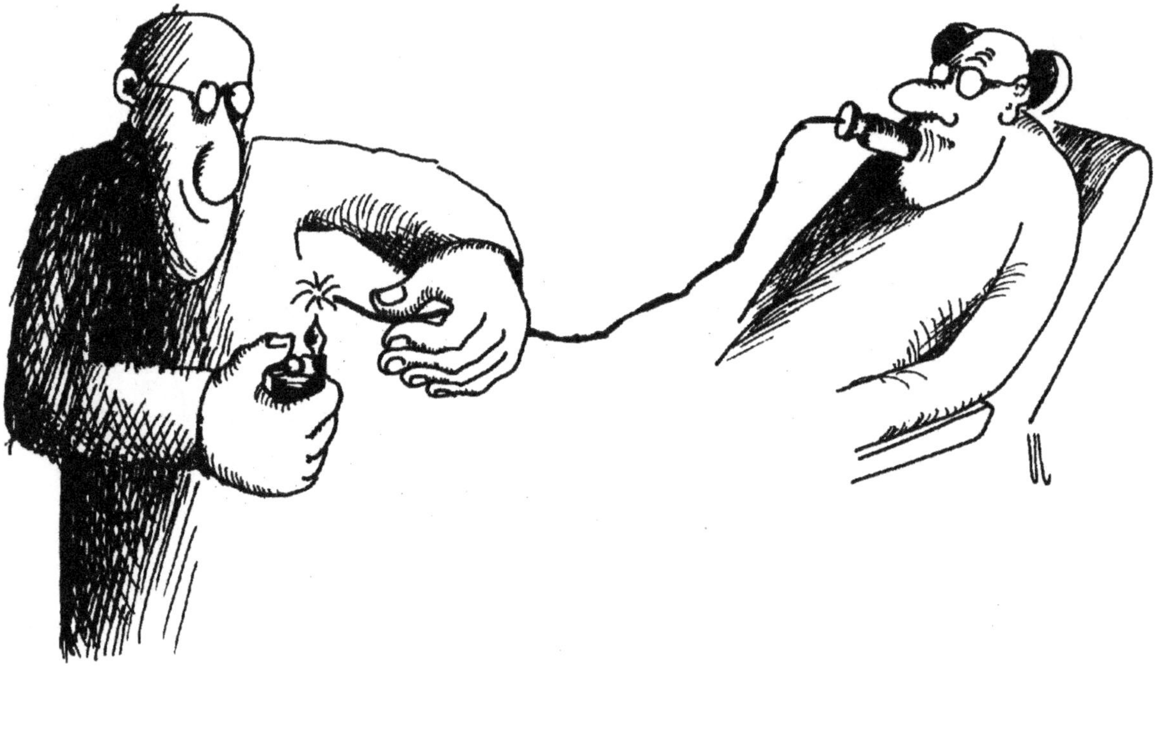

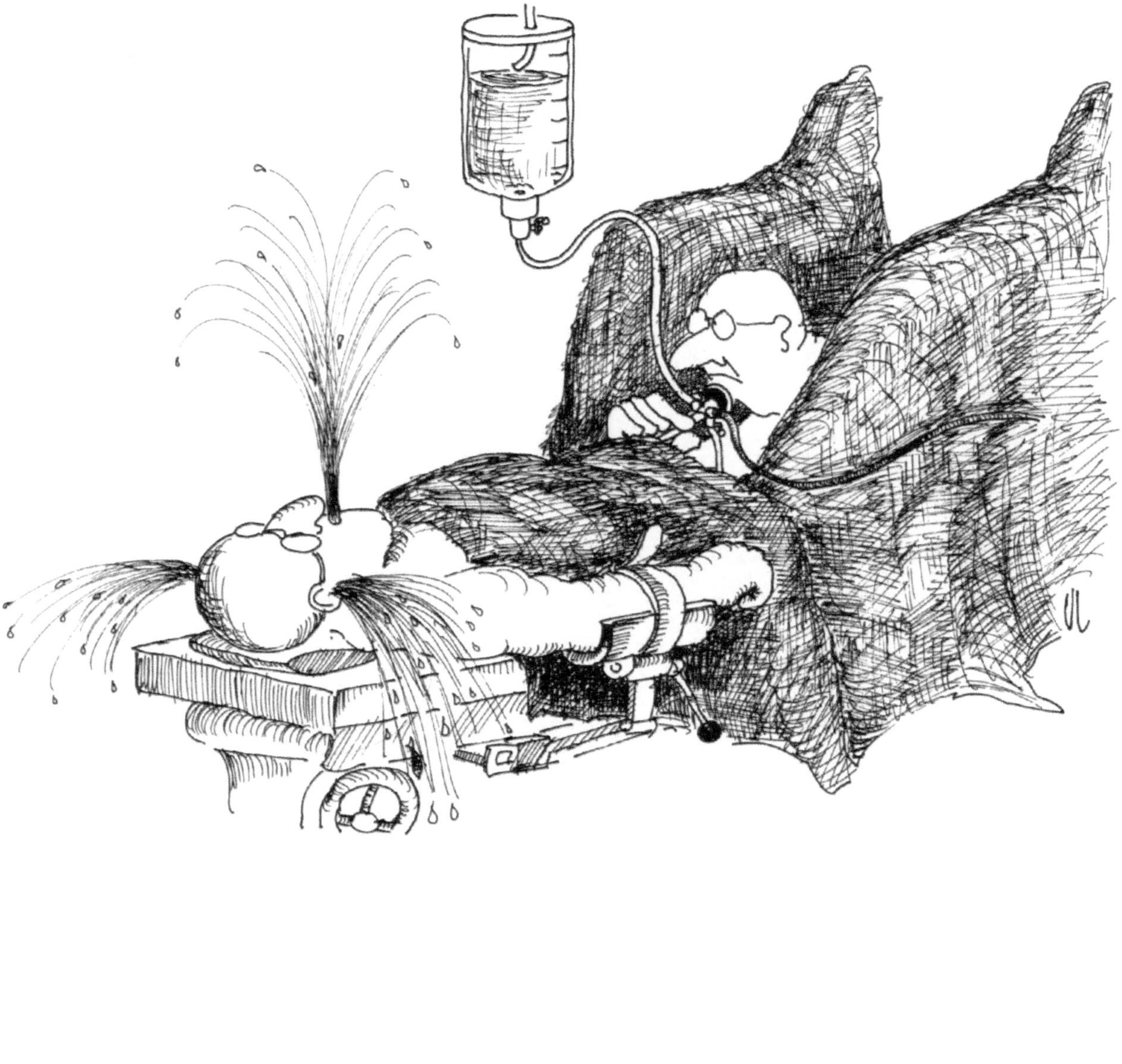

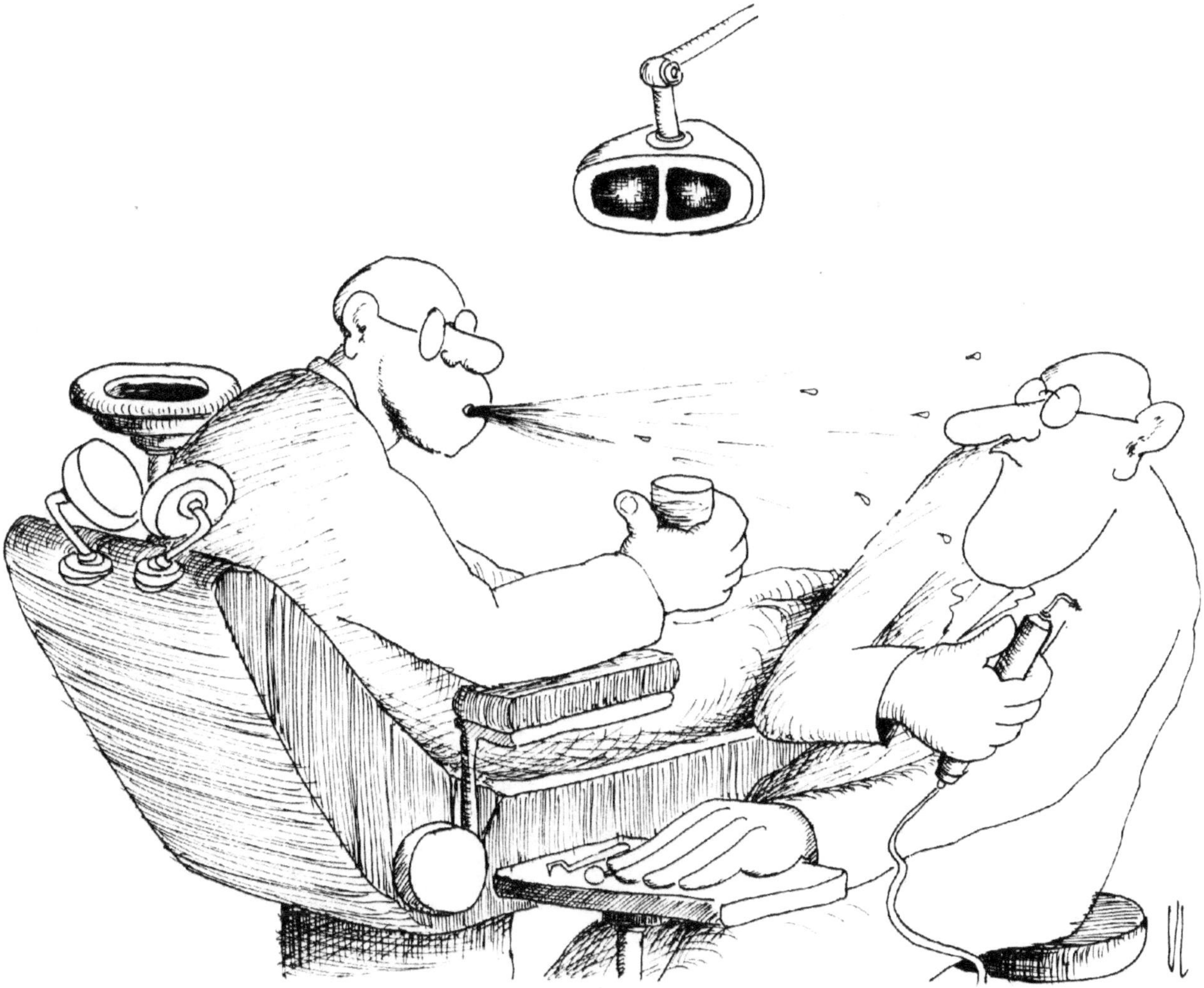

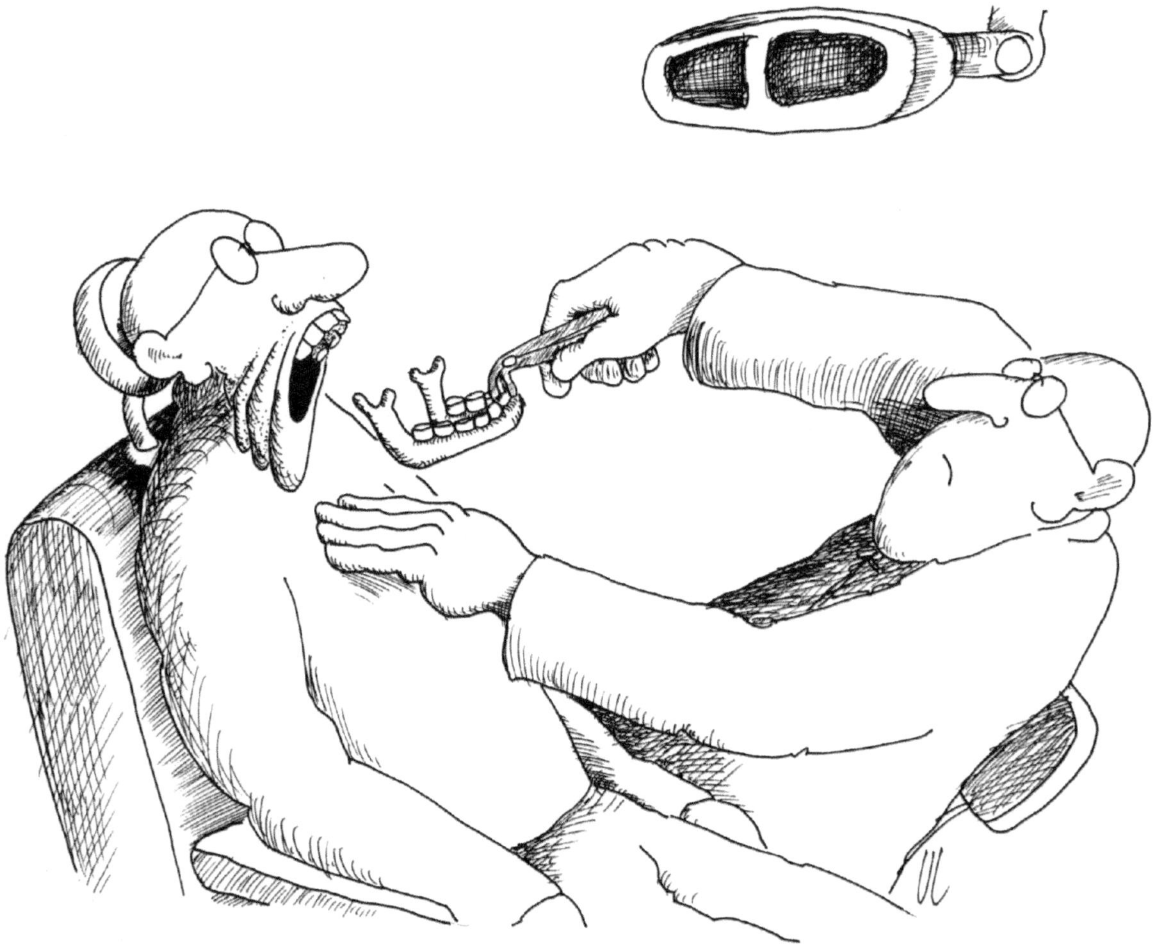

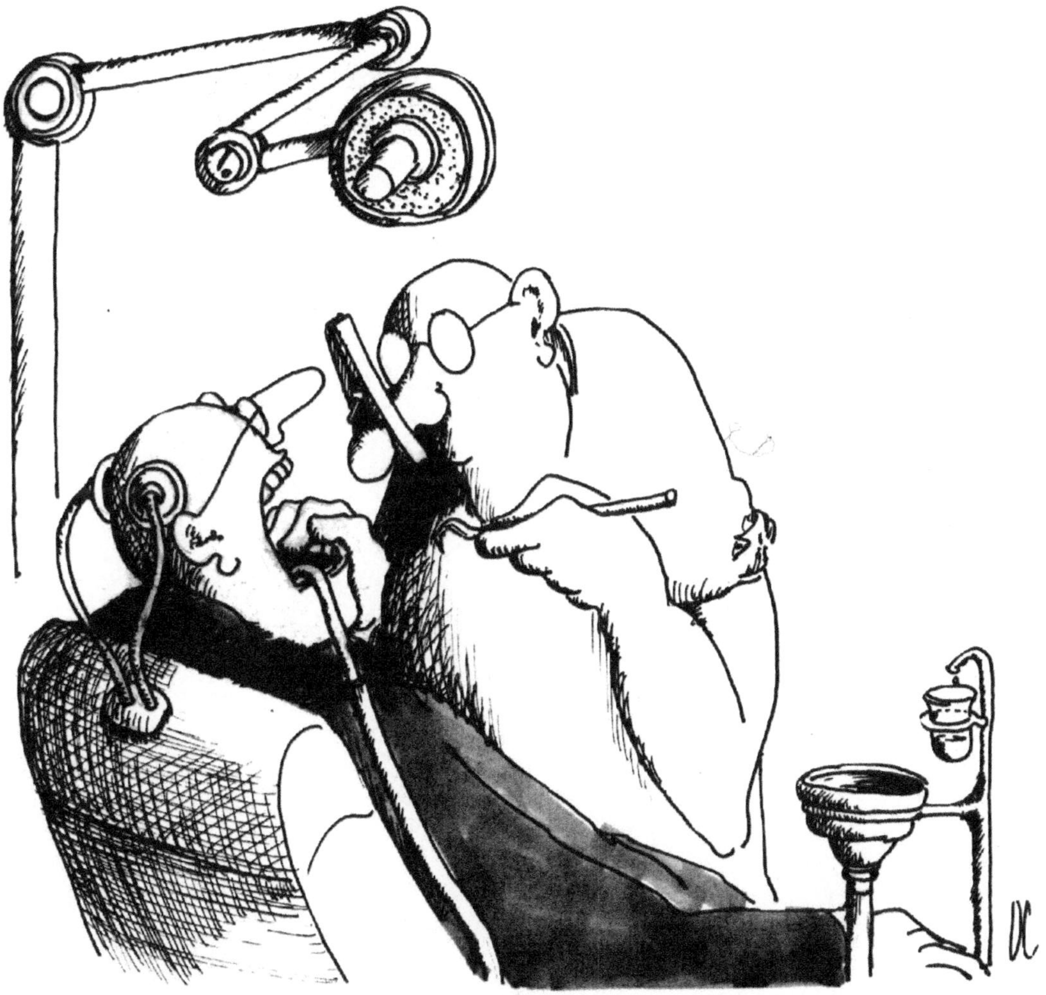

**About the Author**

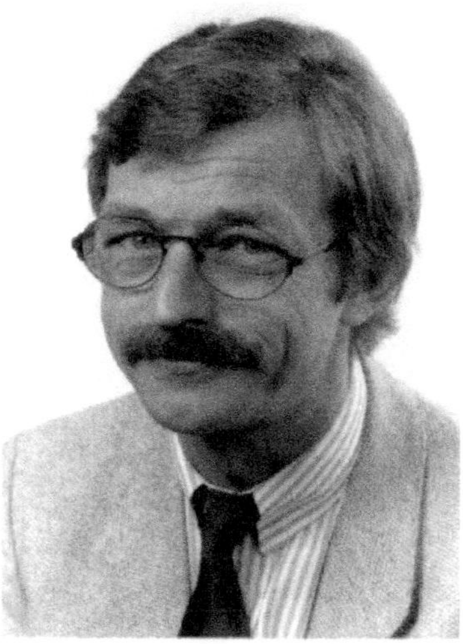

Born 1946 in Kiel, Germany
Medical School in Hamburg, Heidelberg and Lübeck
Exam and Promotion 1973 in Lübeck
Residency in General Surgery in Münster und Lübeck
Attending Physician for Surgery, Traumatology and Vascular Surgery
Assistant Medical Director, Munich-Grosshadern
Head of Surgery at the Schlosspark-Klinik in Berlin since 1993
Married, 3 sons
Hobby Cartoonist

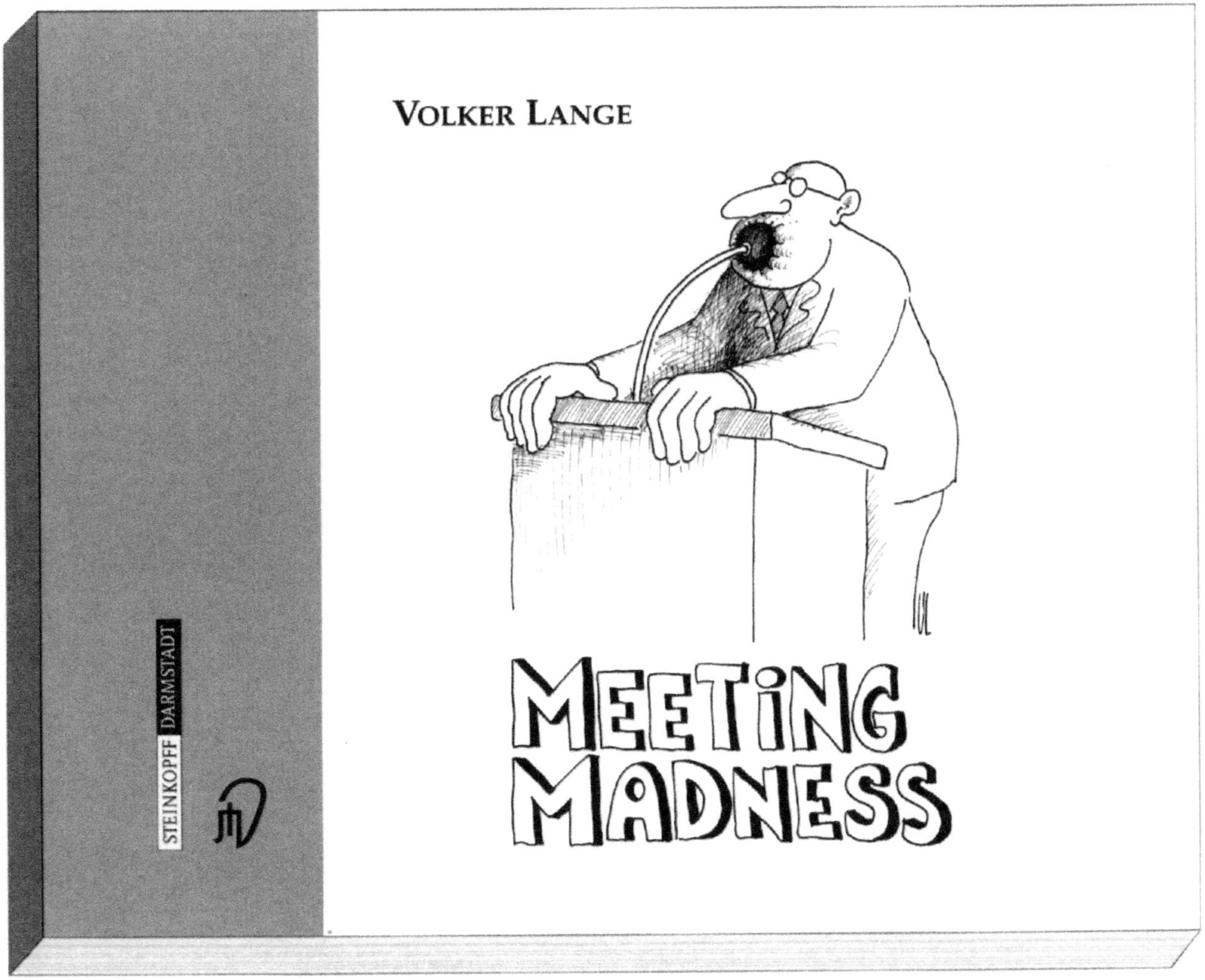
VOLKER LANGE
MEETING MADNESS
STEINKOPFF DARMSTADT

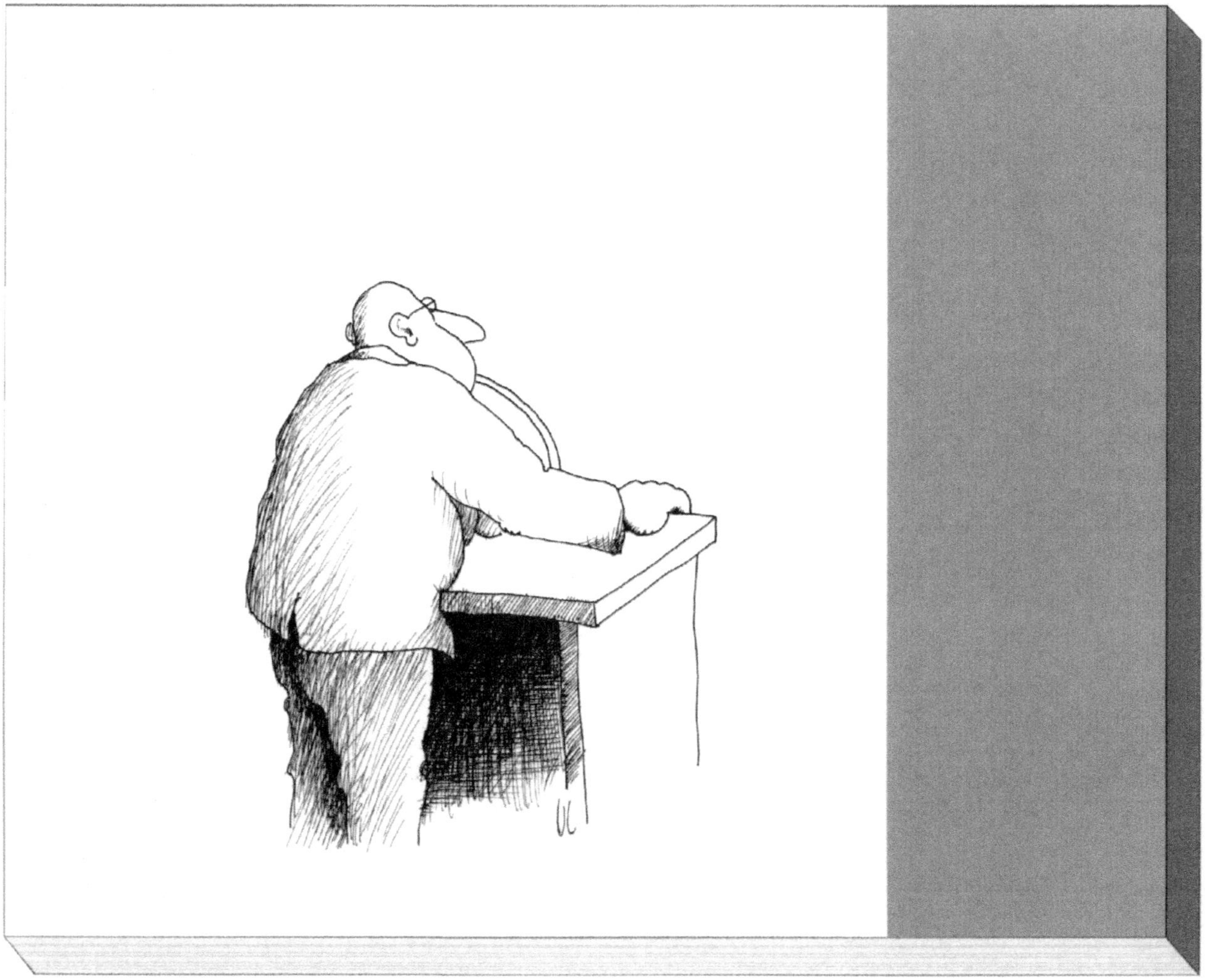

GPSR Compliance

*The European Union's (EU) General Product Safety Regulation (GPSR) is a set of rules that requires consumer products to be safe and our obligations to ensure this.*

*If you have any concerns about our products, you can contact us on ProductSafety@springernature.com*

In case Publisher is established outside the EU, the EU authorized representative is:

Springer Nature Customer Service Center GmbH
Europaplatz 3
69115 Heidelberg, Germany

**Batch number: 10730981**

Printed by Printforce, the Netherlands